A Killer Called Malaria

The Disease That Kills Two People Every Minute

Dr. Kofi Oteng Gyang

authorHOUSE®

AuthorHouse™
1663 Liberty Drive
Bloomington, IN 47403
www.authorhouse.com
Phone: 1-800-839-8640

First published by AuthorHouse 9/21/2009

ISBN: 978-1-4490-1919-8 (sc)

Printed in the United States of America
Bloomington, Indiana

This book is printed on acid-free paper.

A KILLER CALLED MALARIA
The Disease That Kills Two People Every Minute

Kofi Oteng Gyang

Published by the Stop Malaria Now Foundation

MALARIA TABLE OF CONTENTS

Chapter 1: What is malaria? 5
 -Introduction 5
 -Types of Plasmodium parasites that cause Malaria 6
 -Malaria is transmitted by the Anopheles mosquito 8
 -Malaria and other mosquito-borne diseases 10
(Malarias, Filarias, Yellow fever, Dengue, St.Louis
  encephalitis, Eastern Equine encephalitis, Western
 Equine encephalitis, La Crosse encephalitis,
 Japanese encephalitis, West Nile Virus)
 -Malaria deaths in Africa and the World ....`.... 17
Chapter 2: History of the malaria 19
 -History of malaria disease   19
 -Major milestones in discoveries about malaria 23
 -History of malaria treatment   28
Chapter 3: The life cycle of the mosquito 28
 -Breeding places 28
 -Phase of the Mosquito Life Cycle 28
       -Egg phase 29
       -Larva phase 31
       -Pupa phase 31
       -Adult phase 32
 -Some characteristics of adult female mosquitoes
 (Anopheles, Aedes, Culex, Culiseta) 33
Chapter 4: Transmission of the Disease and its Evolution............ 36
 -The Plasmodium parasites 36
 -How the parasites get into humans 40
       -the female mosquito introduces the
          parasites into humans 41
       -sporozoites travel to the human liver
          and multiply 42
       -parasites leave the liver cells and re-enter the
          blood stream 43

-many daughter merozoites are released
into the blood stream 45
-some merozoites change to a sexual stage
(gametocytes) 46
-the gametocytes grow inside the mosquito
and become sporozoites again 46
-Diagnosing malaria 49

Chapter 5: Treatment and Prevention of Malaria 50
-Treatment of Malaria 50
-the Cinchona plant (Quinine) 50
-the *Artemisia annua L.* plant 54
-artemisia and its cultivation 56
-extraction of artemisinin from leaves 57
-Current recommendations for the treatment of:
* *falciparum* malaria 57
* complicated *falciparum* 58
* pregnant women 58
* P. vivax and P. ovale infections 59
* *P. malariae* infections 60
* mixed Plasmodium infections 60
-Other drugs (synthetic drugs and African herbal
preparations) 61
-Diet in the treatment of malaria 62
-Malaria Prevention Drugs... 64
(atovaquone, chloroquine phosphate, doxycycline,
hydroxychloroquine sulfate, mefloquine, primaquine.

Chapter 6: Vector Reduction by Physical Control Methods
-Physical control methods 73
-Bed nets/mosquito nets 75
-Use of screens on house entrances 77
-Use of catch and destroy traps 78
* simple catch and destroy traps 81
* sophisticated catch and destroy traps 86
-Use of sound waves to destroy mosquito larvae 88

Chapter 7: Vector Reduction by Biological and

Chemical Control Methods 90

-Biological control methods..................................... 90

   -use of natural predators 90

   -use of bacteria as larvicides 91

   (Bacillus thuringensis, B, sphaericus)

   -use of fish in ponds 92

   -use of birds, bats, dragonflies and frogs

   that feed on mosquitoes 93

   -use of insect regulator hormones (s-methoprene....... 94

   -the development of an effective vaccine 94

   -the sterilization of male mosquitoes by

   ionizing irradiation............................. 96

-Chemical control methods 96

   -the use of insecticides (generalized spraying) 96

   -the use of insect repellents

   (mosquito coils, skin repellents, etc) 98

Chapter 8: Eradication of Malaria 101

-Malaria control versus malaria eradication 101

-How will eradication be successfully accomplished? 103

-Lessons from the failed malaria eradication project

  in the 1950s 104

-Incorporating vector controls in malaria eradication 105

-Incorporating political, social and economic factors 106

-Management of malaria eradication agencies 115

Chapter 9: Economic Implications of Malaria Eradication 117

-Is malaria eradication possible in developing nations? 118

-Has malaria been eradicated in some developing

  nations? Yes! 118

-Malaria eradication will bring riches to nations................. 119

-Costs of malaria to individuals 120

-Costs of malaria to governments 121

-Tolerating Malaria: a question of misplaced priorities? 122

-Conclusion. 124

References...................................... 125

Chapter 1: WHAT IS MALARIA

INTRODUCTION

Malaria is the most widespread of several diseases caused by mosquitoes. It is estimated that malaria kills a healthy child somewhere in the world every thirty seconds. Several medical records indicate that malaria kills one out of five babies before they reach their fifth birthday. It also very frequently attacks pregnant women, leading to disastrous consequences for the unborn. However, malaria does not prey solely on the weak and vulnerable; it affects and kills many healthy men and women too.

Malaria disease is present in over ninety countries in the world. It adversely affects the daily lives of about 2.4 billion people, which is about 40% of the world's population, reducing the lives of most of them to one of extreme hardship, hopelessness and poverty. Estimated malaria deaths are around two million people a year. About 90% of these deaths from malaria occur in tropical and sub-tropical Africa, although reports indicate that the prevalence of the disease in increasing in Asia and South America. It is significant to note that, in these troubled parts of Africa, young children account for 90% of all malaria deaths.

Malaria is caused by a parasite called *Plasmodium*. This parasite is introduced into a human victim through the blood sucking action of a female mosquito. The parasite then develops in the human being, first in the liver and then in the infected person's red blood cells, leading to significant destruction of these red blood cells in the process. This wanton destruction of the human victim's red blood cells results in fever, headache, joint pains, general weakness and shivering. In the absence of adequate immunity or treatment, the disease continues its course, leading to anemia, spleen enlargement, jaundice, kidney failure, coma and death.

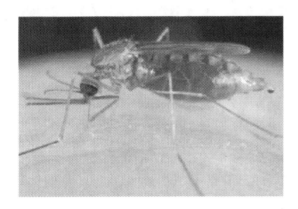

Fig. 1-1: A female mosquito sucks blood from a human victim to develop its eggs. At the same time, it introduces deadly parasites into the human victim (courtesy of CDC).

TYPES OF PLASMODIUM PARASITES THAT CAUSE MALARIA

It is estimated that up to 200 *Plasmodium* parasites may be introduced into a human victim during the process of a single blood sucking action of an infected mosquito. These parasites may be of similar or different species depending on the geographical location of the infection.

In general, there are four different species of Plasmodium parasites capable of infecting human beings. These are:

–*Plasmodium falciparum* mostly found in Africa, New Guinea, Haiti

–*Plasmodium malariae* mostly found in endemic areas in Tropical Africa

–*Plasmodium ovale* mostly found in Africa and Southern India

–*Plasmodium vivax* found in India, South and Central America, Asia and Oceania.

Each of these parasites is carried by a different species of mosquito. In addition, malaria disease resulting from each one of these parasites has slightly different symptoms and characteristics.

Plasmodium falciparum which is prevalent in Tropical Africa causes the most   lethal type of malaria, and the type of malaria most difficult to control.

Plasmodium malariae causes quartan malaria which produces fever, headache and shivering every third day.

Plasmodium ovale causes ovale malaria. It also causes tertian malaria which   produces   fever,   headache   and shivering every other day.

Plasmodium vivax is mostly found in Asia and although not very lethal, it is the   most difficult to cure completely. Vivax malaria rarely affects black Africans due to the absence of a specific factor on the surface of the red blood cells of these Africans, with which the parasite needs to bind. *P. vivax* also causes tertian   malaria which produces fever, headache and shivering every other day.

Treatment modalities for these different types of malaria also vary. For instance, patients treated from malaria due to *Plasmodium malariae, Plasmodium vivax* and *Plasmodium ovale* require a secondary treatment after completion of the primary infection, in order to prevent recurrences of the same treated infection.

African people with sickle cell trait also have relative immunity from severe malaria sickness. A number of people living in endemic regions tend to acquire some limited natural immunity to malaria but this immunity dissipates quickly when they leave the malaria endemic areas.

MALARIA IS CARRIED BY THE ANOPHELES MOSQUITO

Malaria disease is carried from person to person by the Anopheles mosquito. Anopheles mosquitoes are present in all parts of the world except Antarctica but not all of them are carriers of the disease. Malaria carrying Anophelines are present even in countries where malaria has been eradicated and this therefore puts all countries at perpetual risk for re-introduction of the disease.

What are mosquitoes?
The scientific classification of the mosquito is shown below.

Kingdom	Animalia	Animal
Phylum	Arthropoda	Arthropods
Class	Insecta	Insects
Order	Diptera	2 wings
Family	Culicidae	
Genus	Anopheles, Culex, Culiseta, Aedes	

Mosquitoes are flying insects responsible for inflicting tremendous suffering and pain to human beings. They belong to the order Diptera, which are true flying insects with scaly wings. They have long legs, slim bodies and feed mostly on nectar and fruit juice. The male mosquito has a feathery antenna with mouth parts which cannot pierce the human skin. On the other hand the female mosquito has a long, piercing mouthpart called a **proboscis**. The female mosquito uses this proboscis to pierce the human skin in order to suck blood from its victims. This piercing action hurts and often results in painful skin blisters.

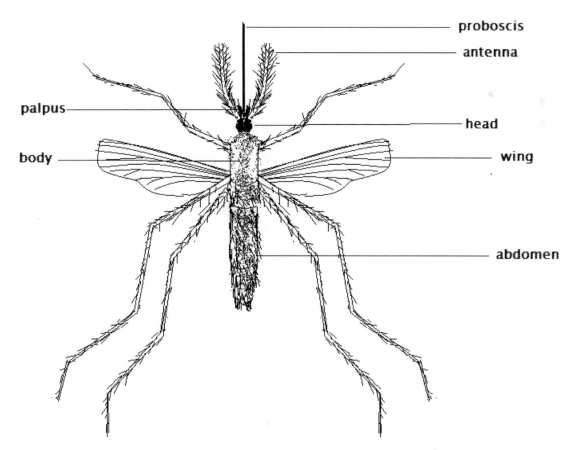

Fig. 1-2: *An adult female mosquito (courtesy Dr. Oteng Gyang)*

As if that is enough, an infected female mosquito injects Plasmodium parasites into its human victims when sucking blood from them. These parasites first develop in the liver, then emerge into the blood stream within a week or two and enter the red blood cells of the human victim. Here they develop and multiply, and burst out occasionally from the red blood cells in large numbers when their populations are high. This process destroys the human victim's red blood cells leading to anemia.

MALARIA AND OTHER MOSQUITO BORNE DISEASES

Many Biologists estimate that there are 2500 to 3500 species of mosquitoes in the world and these are grouped into 41 genera. Of these genera, 430-460 species are Anopheles out of which 30-68 species transmit malaria. These Anopheles species are therefore called **malaria carriers** or **malaria vectors**. These are spread out in all parts of the world. Other mosquito carriers of disease belong to the following genera: **Aedes, Culex** and **Culiseta**.

About 170 species of mosquitoes are found in North America, but different species continue to enter, travel within, migrate, evolve, find new habitats and adapt to conditions in the North American continent.

Mosquito-borne diseases

There are 2 main types of mosquito-borne diseases. These are:
-**mosquito-borne protozoan diseases and**
-**mosquito-borne viral diseases.**

...mosquito-borne protozoan diseases

Mosquito borne protozoan diseases are those in which the disease causing organisms carried by the mosquito happen to be protozoa. These include malaria and filaria diseases.

....mosquito borne viral diseases

Mosquito borne viral diseases are those in which the disease causing organisms carried by the mosquito happen to be viruses. These include Yellow fever, Dengue and a variety of encephalites the most important of which are St. Louis encephalitis, Eastern Equine encephalitis, La Crosse encephalitis, Japanese encephalitis and West Nile Virus disease.

Mosquito-borne protozoan diseases: Malarias and Filarias

Malaria

Malaria is caused by a parasite called Plasmodium which is carried by the Anopheles mosquito. Filarias are caused by parasitic worms.

Filaria

A type of filaria disease, also called Canine heartworm is caused by a roundworm called *Dirofilaria immitis*. It is transmitted through the bite of a mosquito. It infects dogs, cats and raccoons. The disease is found in the USA and Canada.

Mosquito borne viral diseases: Yellow fever, Dengue and the Encephalites

Mosquito borne viral diseases include Yellow fever, Dengue, a variety of encephalites.

Mosquito –borne Protozoan parasitic diseases

Types of disease	Mosquito carrier	Type of parasite / virus
Malaria	Anopheles sp.	Plasmodium falciparum
Filaria (dog roundworm)		Dirofilaria immitis

Mosquito borne Virus diseases

Types of disease	Mosquito carrier	Type of parasite / virus
Yellow fever		Arboviral
Dengue	Aedes aegypti,	Arboviral
	Aedes albopictus	Arboviral
Encephalitis		
-St. Louis Encephalitis	Culex spp.	Arboviral
	Culex pipiens	Flavivirus
-Eastern Equine Encephalitis	Culex spp,	Arboviral
	Culiseta melanura	Arboviral
-Western Equine Encephalitis	Culex tarsalis	
-LaCrosse Encephalitis	Aedes triseriatus	
-Japanese Encephalitis		
-West Nile Virus.	Culex pipiens	Flavivirus

Table 1-1: Diseases which are carried by mosquitoes.

Yellow Fever

Yellow fever is an extremely infectious disease caused by an arbovirus which lives in monkeys without any apparent effect on these monkeys. It is transmitted to humans through the bite of the mosquito *Aedes aegypti* which also gets it from an infected monkey when it bites the monkey for a blood meal. There are five marked stages in Yellow fever infection. The third stage called intoxication can lead to degeneration of the affected persons internal organs especially the heart, kidney and liver. The eyes of the infected person turn yellow and he/she may throw out blood as black vomit. Proteins accumulate in the kidney as the kidney functions shut down. Many deaths follow this stage.

The history of yellow fever is filled with several cases of human deaths in many areas of the world. For example, in Cuba, in the 1760's, the disease killed thousands of American and English troops who had invaded the island. Also, in mainland United States, in 1793, Yellow fever sent about 10% of all of Philadelphia's citizens to their graves. In Haiti, in 1902, when the French Emperor Napoleon sent forty thousand soldiers to fight African slaves seeking their freedom, Yellow fever fought on the side of the poor Africans led by Toussaint L'Ouverture, and helped to snuff out the lives of about 30 000 French soldiers. Again in mainland America, in 1855, no less than three thousand Virginians in Norfolk in the United States lost their lives to Yellow fever. In 1878, in the city of Memphis, Tennessee in the Southern United States, the disease was again responsible for the deaths of approximately five thousand people. In West Africa, Yellow fever killed European colonists in their thousands during the era of European colonization of Africa in the 19th century, thus earning for this African coast the unenviable reputation of 'the white man's grave.'

Today, Yellow fever is still a dreaded disease with an estimated 200 000 reported cases in 33 different countries of the world every year. These infections result in 30 000 deaths worldwide. Twenty seven deaths from Yellow fever were reported in the southern Sudan in 2003 and 99 in the

Americas. One Yellow fever death was reported in the USA in 2002.

Dengue

Dengue is an arboviral disease caused by a virus which is carried by *Aedes aegypti* and *Aedes albopictus* mosquitoes. Dengue disease is characterized by hemorrhages, and fever of the infected individual and may result in death. Its presence has been reported in practically all parts of the world but more importantly in Brazil (350 000 cases in 2002 with 42 deaths), India, Bangladesh, Asia, North and South America and Africa. In 2002, 54 000 cases were reported in Indonesia with over 600 deaths.

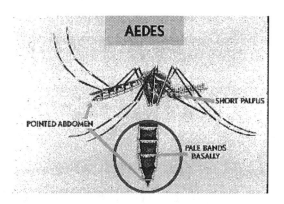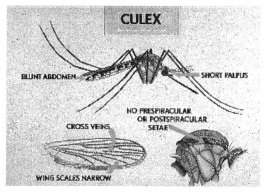

Fig. 1-3: Aedes mosquitoes are characterized by a pointed abdomen, short palpus, and pale bands at the base of each abdomen. The Culex mosquito (right) is characterized by a blunt abdomen, cross veins on narrow wings, short palpus and no prespiracular or postspiraclular septae (courtesy CDC).

St Louis encephalitis

St Louis encephalitis is caused by a virus whose vector is the *Culex* mosquito. The disease targets mainly children and the elderly. St. Louis encephalitis occurs in the United States especially in Florida and along the Gulf Coast but cases have been reported in the Western United States (California) too in 1997. Chicken infections were also reported in 2003 in California in the USA. There is no vaccine for St. Louis encephalitis.

Eastern Equine Encephalitis

Eastern Equine Encephalitis is transmitted by *Culiseta melanura* and other Culex species. It affects humans and horses in North America, South America and the Caribbean islands. Symptoms include none to a mild flu with fever, headaches and sore throat. Some infections result in serious complications that affect the Central nervous system. Such serious infections result in sudden fever and headaches leading to seizures, coma and death. About 50% of patients who get serious complications from this infection die from the disease. Those who survive end up with permanent brain damage and become incapacitated for life. There is no treatment for Eastern Equine Encephalitis. A vaccine is available for horses but not for human beings. Of the 8 cases reported in the USA in 2003, four of the infected patients died.

Western Equine Encephalitis

Western Equine encephalitis is caused by a virus that is carried by the mosquito *Culex tarsalis*. It was first found in a horse in 1930. Birds and small mammals are hosts. It is non specific in humans. A vaccine has been developed for horses but none is available for humans.

LaCrosse Encephalitis

Lacrosse encephalitis got its name from the town where it was first recorded I n 1963, LaCrosse, Wisconsin in the USA. It is caused by a virus that is carried by a type of woodland mosquito called *Aedes triseriatus*. This mosquito is also called the tree hole mosquito. LaCrosse encephalitis affects young children below the age of 16. it is mainly found in the USA east of the Mississippi river. There is no vaccine for Lacrosse encephalitis.

Japanese encephalitis

Japanese encephalitis is predominant in Japan where about 50 000 cases are reported every year.

West Nile Virus

West Nile Virus is caused by a Flavivirus which is also transmitted by a variety of mosquitoes. The most common species of mosquito implicated in human and horse infections belongs to the *Culex pipiens* group.

West Nile virus disease has been reported in North America, Africa, Europe and the Middle East. People infected with mild West Nile Virus infections may show flu-like symptoms, including fever, headache, tiredness, aches or a rash. Other types of West Nile virus diseases attack the nervous system leading to swelling of the brain and the membranes around it.

Several cases of West Nile virus disease have been reported in New York in the USA. In 1999, sixty-two confirmed cases of West Nile virus were reported in New York; seven of these patients died. In 2001, of the sixty-six human cases reported in New York, ten of the patients died. In 2002, a total of almost four thousand human cases were reported with over two hundred and thirty deaths. There is a West Nile Virus vaccine for horses but none for humans.

Malaria deaths in Africa and the world

Conservative estimates put the yearly death toll from malaria alone between one million and two million every year in the world but the real numbers may be higher than these estimates. This is because the disease is endemic and prevalent in poor areas of the world where autopsy statistics are not a national priority and are therefore not readily available. Moreover, when some of these people who have been persistently weakened by malaria die as a result of other opportunistic infections, their deaths are never attributed to malaria.

There are 3 main ways malaria kills children in Africa. Malaria may infect a child directly and quickly, leading to a devastating and highly acute infection with seizures, cerebral malaria, coma and death. Secondly, continuous and persistent malaria may debilitate a child, leading to persistent weakness and anemia with reduced body inability to fight off other infections leading to increased risk of loss of life. Finally, malaria infected pregnant women with poor health may give birth to children with low birth weight. In such cases, death of the newborn may occur within 30 days after birth.

In the case of adults, malaria consistently weakens the body's physique, rendering the individuals concerned continuously weak and unhealthy as it infects and re-infects them even after treatment. This process of infection and reinfection renders these individuals susceptible to other diseases and robs them of important financial resources as well as the necessary peace of mind required to realize their full potential. This leads to a cycle of poverty and disillusionment for hundreds of millions of people.

Chapter 2:	HISTORY OF MALARIA

HISTORY OF MALARIA DISEASE

The name malaria comes from two Italian words corrupted into *mal'aria* which means 'bad air. This name was coined in the seventh century B.C.E. to describe a disease which was prevalent in foul-smelling swampy areas near Rome, the capital city of the Roman Empire during that time. However the disease was known long before the seventh century B.C.E.

.....*ancient Chinese writings described malaria fever*

Ancient Chinese medical literature, the *Nei Ching*, which dates from 2700 BCE and which was edited by the then Chinese Emperor Huang Ti, documents a disease with the characteristic symptoms of the malaria disease.

.......*ancient Hindu literature attributes malaria to the bites of certain insects*

Some researchers have found accounts of the disease in Vedic writings in India going back 3600 years. Ancient Sanskrit medical literature, the *Susruta*, described the symptoms of malaria disease and recorded that it was due to the bites of certain insects.

...*Hippocrates described malaria..*

In the fifth century B.C.E., the Greek scientist and physician, Hippocrates described the disease and found a relationship between its outbreaks and the seasons. Of course, epidemics occurred more during the wet and warmer periods of the year. Large outbreaks of malaria epidemics at the time were reported to be responsible for the decline of many city-state populations in several areas of what is now modern-day Greece.

....did malaria bring about the fall of Rome?

Other scientific texts have revealed the presence of malaria in the bones of a child who died 1500 years ago and was buried near Rome. The evidence from this child's corpse also suggests that malaria epidemics occurred during the hey-days of the Roman Empire long before the Christian era. Due to the prevalent nature of malaria at the time, some researchers believe that malaria may have played a major role in the fall of the Roman Empire. They suggest that a large epidemic, at some later time, could have made the Roman soldiers too weak to fight forcefully against the Vandals, the Huns and the Visigoths who brought the Roman Empire to its knees.

...disease was prevalent in Europe, Africa, Asia and America

History reveals that malaria disease has been prevalent in Europe, Africa and America for several centuries. It was carried from place to place by invading armies, merchants, missionaries and colonial settlers.

....disease ravaged America before the era of slavery...

Four hundred years of slave trade between Africa and the Americas may have led to its increased transport between the two continents but there is little doubt that malaria was present in America before the era of the slave trade. Historical accounts reveal that in 1607, malaria ruined the Jamestown colony set up by early European settlers in America. During the years that followed, there were regular epidemics in the Southern and Midwestern states until it peaked in 1875. It is believed that by 1914 when the First World War began, over 600 000 new cases of malaria infections were being discovered annually in the United States of America. During the American civil war, over a million cases of malaria were recorded by both the Northern forces and the Confederate armies.

.......malaria nearly killed an American President..

History has it that one United States President John Adams while on a mission to Amsterdam contracted malaria and nearly died.

... the ravages of malaria during the Panama canal construction

In the early 1900s, construction of the Panama Canal was begun. 1n 1906, there were over 26 000 workers at the construction site in Panama. Of these, over 21 000 (80.8%) fell ill and were hospitalized at one time or another. The causes of the diseases which were ravaging the health of these workers were malaria and yellow fever. It must be remembered that the United States had occupied Cuba and Panama at the time. To prevent the collapse of the Panama Canal project, the Americans made great efforts to control the disease. Their efforts were partially successful. By 1912, out of over 50 000 workers, the number of sick, hospitalized workers had fallen dramatically to 5 600 (11.2%). Continued efforts led to the complete elimination of yellow fever and dramatic reduction in the cases of malaria infection and disease.

....malaria in the United States..

In 1914, the United States Congress provided funds to their nation's Public Health Service (USPHS) to control malaria disease in the United States. The USPHS organized malaria control programs in all parts of the country, especially in the warm areas of the Southern United States where malaria was endemic. Substantial efforts were made to reduce mosquito breeding sites through insecticide applications and the control of waterways. These efforts succeeded and enabled military bases in the Southern US to remain open for military training all year round.

Despite their laudable efforts however, by 1933, malaria disease still affected 30% of the United States population, especially in the Tennessee Valley region. It was then that, in May 1933, President Roosevelt signed the US Tennessee Valley Authority bill. It enabled the creation of a centralized body to develop the region through the creation of waterways, land improvement systems and the harnessing of the Tennessee River's potential for hydro-electric purposes. By 1947, with the help of this bill and the efforts of the US Public Health Service, malaria disease was practically eliminated from the United States .

....malaria was a problem during the two World wars, the Korean War and the Vietnam War.

Malaria affected and killed many people during the First World War which was fought in1914-1918. Malaria continued to weaken soldiers and civilians during the Second World War in 1939-1945. The Korean and Vietnam wars were no exception; many soldiers and civilians succumbed to malaria during the period of these wars. Historians and Epidemiologists suggest that a more deadly and drug resistant form of malaria disease appeared during the Vietnam War. It is certainly true that many Americans got infected with malaria disease in both Korea and Vietnam and brought the disease home with them during and after the war.

Major milestones in discoveries concerning the malaria disease

.....in 1880, Dr. Laveran discovers the malaria parasite in human blood in Africa

On October 20 1880, Dr. Charles Laveran, a French Army doctor based in Constantine, Algeria in North Africa, discovered the presence of some crescent-shaped bodies in the blood of one of his patients. This patient was suffering from malaria. These crescent- shaped bodies were all transparent except for the presence of a small pigment dot in them. On further examination of blood samples from about 190 malaria patients, Dr. Laveran identified the same crescent shaped bodies in 148 of these patients. These crescent shaped bodies proved to be the four different stages of the malaria parasite in human blood. Dr. Laveran thought that there was only one species of the malaria parasite and called it *Oscillaria malariae.* The French Army Doctor subsequently received the Nobel Prize for this work which proved to be the stages of the life cycle of the malaria parasite in human blood.

.........in 1886, Golgi finds that there are different malaria parasites and different types of malaria diseases

In 1886, an Italian Neurophysiologist called Camillo Golgi observed that there were at least two forms of malaria disease. These were:

-tertian malaria: which produced fever every second day (every other day)

-quartan malaria: which produced fever every third day. Camillo Golgi also discovered that these different fevers produced different numbers of new parasites (called merozoites) and that the production of fever in the patient coincided with the break up of blood cells and the release of new parasites into the blood stream. Golgi's work won him the Nobel Prize for Neurophysiology in 1906.

........in 1890, 1897, the name Plasmodium is introduced to describe malaria parasites

In 1890, two Italian Scientists, Giovanni Grassi and Raimondo Filetti introduced the name *Plasmodium* to describe two of the parasites responsible for malaria disease: *Plasmodium vivax and Plasmodium malariae*. Later in the decade, 1897, William Welch, an American Scientist named the parasite responsible for tertian malaria disease as *Plasmodium falciparum*. It was not until 1922, that another Scientist called William Stephens described the fourth parasite as *Plasmodium ovale*.

........In 1897, Dr. Ronald Ross demonstrates that mosquitoes transmit malaria

In August 1897, an Indian born British officer, Dr. Ross, demonstrated that malaria parasites could be transmitted from infected patients to mosquitoes. He also showed that mosquitoes could transmit malaria parasites from a sick bird to a healthy one. This revelation proved how malaria transmission occurred. It showed that for malaria disease to infect a healthy person, there was the need for a parasite development stage inside the mosquito. This parasite development stage inside the mosquito is called the *sporogonic* stage. Dr. Ronald Ross received the Nobel Prize for this important discovery in 1902.

....In 1898–1899, Italians show the presence of human malaria parasites

In 1898–1899, Italian scientists confirmed the work of Dr. Ross in human patients. Their work showed that mosquitoes transmit malaria the same way as they do in birds. These scientists collected some live mosquito species of the *Anopheles claviger* species and allowed them to feed on sick, malaria patients in Rome. These well fed, infected mosquitoes were then sent to London where they were made to feed again on two healthy volunteers. Of course, both of the London volunteers developed tertian malaria. This work demonstrated the complete cycle of malaria transmission in humans.

History of malaria treatment

All over the world, there are both written and oral accounts that document human efforts to deal with the scourge of malaria disease. Chinese written records show that in the second century BCE, a plant called Qinghao was used to treat malaria fevers. In the Americas, long before the arrival of the European colonizers, a plant bark found in Peru was used to treat malaria. Later Europeans called this tree bark Peruvian bark. It was not until the Indians taught the newly arrived Europeans its use, and subsequently used it to treat the wife of a Peruvian colonizer called Chinchon was the name abandoned and replaced with Cinchona to reflect the name of the treated Countess.

.....chloroquine was discovered by a German called Hans Andersag

In 1934, a German called Hans Andersag, synthesized chloroquine at Bayer Laboratories in Eberfield, Germany. He called his new compound **resochin**. During and after the Second World War, this compound was re-named chloroquine by American and British scientists.

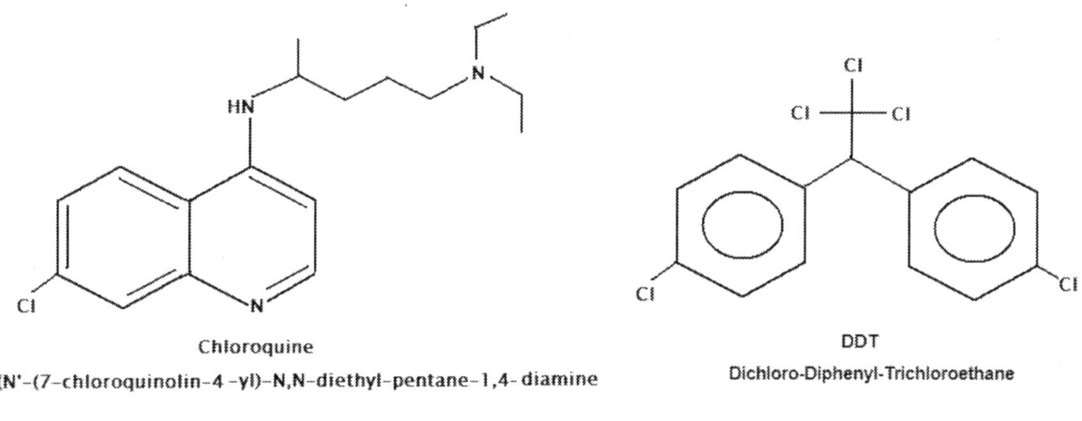

Chloroquine
(N'-(7-chloroquinolin-4-yl)-N,N-diethyl-pentane-1,4-diamine

DDT
Dichloro-Diphenyl-Trichloroethane

Fig. 2-1: Chemical structures of chloroquine (left) and DDT (right).

Fig. 2-1: Chemical structures of chloroquine and DDT.

By 1946, chloroquine was widely known and used to treat malaria effectively in several parts of the world. We shall look at the different chloroquine derivatives as well as other anti-malarial drugs in a later chapter on malaria treatment.

...DDT was synthesized in 1939 by Othmer Zeidler and Paul Muller noticed DDT could kill insects effectively......

It was a German scientist, Othmer Zeidler, who synthesized DDT in 1874. He was preparing his doctorate thesis in Chemistry at the time.

However, it was not until 1939 that a Swiss national, Paul Muller, discovered that DDT could kill insects effectively. At the end of the Second World War, there was widespread use of DDT against insect pests worldwide, notably for malaria control. By 1955, the use of DDT as an insecticide had been found to be so successful that it helped lead world wide efforts to eradicate malaria. By 1962, however, a group of environmentalists in the United States, noticing its toxic side-effects, started to campaign against its indiscriminate and widespread use in North America. In 1972, as a result of their campaign, the use of DDT was banned in North America and subsequently in all other parts of the World under the Stockholm Convention. With this ban, came the collapse of the World Health Organization's world-wide efforts to eradicate malaria disease.

Chapter 3: THE LIFE CYCLE OF THE MOSQUITO

Many mosquitoes live in the wild where they regularly feed on nectars from flowers. They breed, live and die where they hatch. However many females mosquitoes travel long distances in search of blood. It is only the female mosquito which feeds on blood. The female mosquito uses the blood she sucks from human beings, birds and other mammals to fertilize her eggs. But by sucking blood from humans, it secretes mosquito saliva infected with parasites and viruses into the human blood leading to diseases, some of which are fatal to man.

Breeding places

Mosquitoes breed in standing waters. They can breed in fresh water or salt water. Pools, marshes, lakes and slow running streams can all serve as breeding grounds for mosquitoes. Similarly, standing water in old tires, in tree holes and in disused swimming pools constitute favorable areas for mosquito proliferation.

Phases of the mosquito life cycle

The mosquito has four distinct life cycles. These are:
-Egg phase
-Larva phase
-Pupa phase
-Adult mosquito phase

During each phase, the growing mosquito shows a special appearance with different characteristics.

Step 1   : Egg stage

The female mosquito lays her eggs on the surface of stagnant water. Mosquito eggs are light and float on the surface of the water. As has already been noted, any pool of water that collects in tins, cans, ditches, gutters, lorry tires especially after a rainfall can serve as a breeding place. Pools of permanent, stagnant water like swamps, or slow flowing streams may also be used to serve this purpose. In slow flowing streams and rivers, the female mosquitoes will usually lay her eggs in areas sheltered from wind by overgrown weeds or grass.

In the case of the *Anopheles* and *Aedes* species, the eggs are laid one at a time and remain in the water in singles. The Anopheles mosquito's single egg has floats on the sides which help it to remain on top of the water and prevent it from sinking.

In the case of the *Culex* and *Culiseta* species, the eggs are laid singly and then stuck together by the mosquito in rafts of 200 to 300 on the surface of the water. These rafts of eggs are usually dark colored and measure about 0.6cm long by 0.3cm wide. A *Culex* mosquito may lay a raft of eggs every three nights during its life span.

Compared to the other mosquitoes, the *Culiseta* mosquito does not lay her eggs on stagnant water but in damp soil in an area where it will later be flooded. However, like the *Culex* species of mosquito, the *Culiseta* eggs are also laid singly and then stuck together by the mosquito in rafts of 200 to 300.

It is believed that an adult female mosquito may lay a total of 1000 – 3000 eggs during its lifetime.

Species	Where eggs are laid	Form of the eggs
Anopheles	water	they float singly
Aedes	damp soil	they are laid singly; later flooded by water
Culex	water	they are held together in hundreds like rafts
Culiseta	water	they are held together in hundreds like rafts

Table 3-1: Some characteristics of Mosquito eggs

Most eggs hatch and change to larvae within 48 hours. The Aedes mosquito eggs hatch only when flooded with water from overflowing streams or high tides.

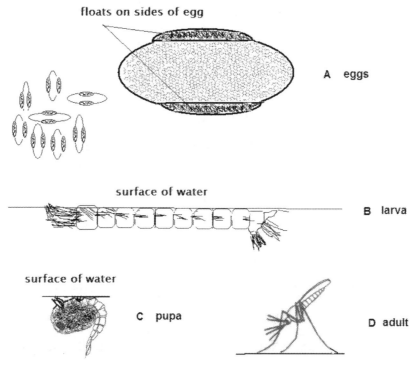

Fig. 3-1: Stages of the life cycle of the Anopheles mosquito. (Diagram by Dr. Oteng Gyang)

Step 2: Larva stage

Under favorable conditions of temperature, humidity and the presence of water, the eggs hatch within 48 hours and tiny larvae emerge. These are called 'wigglers' because they are like little worms and they wiggle when the water surface is disturbed. The larvae feed on algae, organic mater and microorganisms in the water.

These larvae live in the water but need oxygen from above the water surface to breathe. Therefore, the Anopheles larva aligns its body parallel to the surface of the water breathing through a "breathing opening" on its side. Other larvae have a tube on the head called a "siphon" through which they breathe. These larvae may hang from the surface of the water with this siphon.

The larvae hold on to the surface by means of the water surface tension. Any action that leads to breaking this surface tension makes the larvae sink and drown. Surface tension on water may be broken by a drop of oil or kerosene on the water surface.

The larva sheds its skin four times during this stage, while growing bigger and bigger each time. The stage of skin shedding is called "molting." The period between the times when the larva sheds its skin is called "instar." At the time of the 4th instar, the larva measures about 1.2 – 1.3 cm in length. On the fourth molt, a pupa emerges.

Step 3: Pupa stage

As indicated above, after the 4th molt, a pupa emerges. The pupa hangs on to the surface of the water, because it needs oxygen to breathe. At this stage, it breathes through two tubes called 'trumpets' that are located on the large head.

Here again, the pupa holds on to the surface of the water by means of the surface tension of the water. Again, breaking the surface tension leads to sinking, drowning and subsequent death of the pupa.

The pupa does not eat. It moves about and swims in the water though it may also, sometimes, hang quietly on the surface of the water. However, when the water surface is disturbed, it moves in a jerking motion down the water but immediately re-surfaces to hang on to the surface again.

Step 4: Adult mosquito stage

Depending on the type of mosquito, the pupa becomes an adult mosquito within a period of 1-4 days. At the appropriate time, the skin of the pupa splits and the adult mosquito emerges. This new adult mosquito will rest on the surface of the water for a little while in order for its wings to dry and its body to become hard. It then flies away, becoming one more pest that human beings have to deal with.

In general therefore, it takes about 10 to 14 days for a mosquito egg to change into an adult mosquito. Temperature plays a leading role in the duration of this life cycle of the mosquito. At higher temperatures, the process is shortened. For example, the culex mosquito species, *Culex tarsalis*, found in California goes through this cycle in 14 days at 21° C. (70°

F). However, at an increased temperature of 27o C (80 o F), the period of its life cycle is shortened to 10 days.

Average life span of the mosquito

The average life span of the mosquito varies from 3 to 100 days. The male may live from 10 to 20 days. The life span of the female mosquito is much longer and may last from 3 to 100 days depending on the species and genera.

Some characteristics of female adult mosquitoes

The *Anopheles gambiae* and the *Anopheles funestus*, both found in Tropical Africa are some of the most dangerous malaria carriers. This is because they live for a relatively long time, feed preferentially on human beings and hang around human dwellings. They bite at all times, but mostly at dusk, at dawn or during the night.

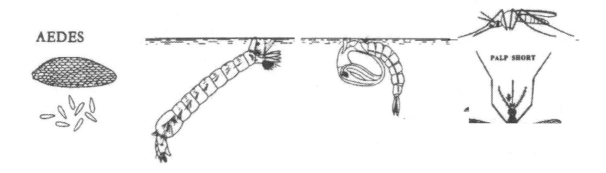

Fig. 3-2: Life cycle of the Aedes mosquito. Note the low sitting position of the abdomen of the adult. The eggs are held together in rafts, the larva hangs, head down, transversally from the water surface (courtesy CDC)

Aedes mosquitoes are painful and persistent biters. They attack during the day but not at night. Aedes mosquitoes do not enter houses or human dwellings. They are very strong fliers and can be found several miles away from their original breeding places.

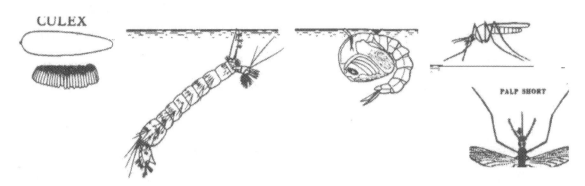

Fig. 3-3: Life cycle of the Culex mosquito. Like the Aedes, the eggs are stuck together in rafts and the larva hangs transversally down from the water surface. The adult in the sitting position has its abdomen parallel to the resting surface (courtesy CDC).

Culex mosquitoes are aggressive and persistent biters. They lay their eggs at night. In addition, they stay in the shade during the day and attack from the period when the sun goes down. They enter houses and human dwellings easily and frequently in search of human blood. Culex mosquitoes are considered weak fliers but reports have found some of them about two miles from their breeding places.

Culiseta mosquitoes attack in the shade during the day, or in the open when the sun goes down. They are reported to be moderately aggressive biters.

.....Mosquitoes in temperate regions

In temperate climates, mosquitoes hibernate during the cold months of the year. They emerge and multiply mostly during the warm months of the year. Those that emerge during late summer in temperate and cold regions of the world may live for a few weeks and then search for sheltered areas to hibernate until spring.

Malaria and a host of other terrible diseases that afflict man and domestic animals are transmitted by mosquitoes. The breaking of the life cycle of the mosquito can lead to the disappearance of these terrible afflictions and help human beings in several countries lead better and prosperous lives. Let us act now to break this cycle.

Remember! No mosquito, No malaria!

Chapter 4: MALARIA TRANSMISSION AND DISEASE EVOLUTION

The Plasmodium parasite

Malaria disease is caused by a parasite called **Plasmodium**. A parasite is an organism that lives in or feeds on another organism, taking whatever it wants and not giving anything useful back. A parasite may even produce toxins inside the host organism thus poisoning it and eventually destroying it.

The scientific classification of the Plasmodium parasite is shown below.

Kingdom: Protista
Phylum: Apicomplexa
Class   Aconoidasida
Order: Haemosporida
Family: Plasmodiidae
Genus: Plasmodium
Species: P. falciparum, P. vivax. P. malariae, P. ovale

There are four species of Plasmodium parasites that infect humans and cause malaria. These are *Plasmodium falciparum*, *P. vivax*, *P. malariae* and *P. ovale.*
These Plasmodium parasites cause different types of malaria:
–*Plasmodium falciparum* is responsible for falciparum malaria or malignant malaria.
–*Plasmodium vivax* is responsible for tertian and vivax malaria
–*Plasmodium malariae* is responsible for quartan malaria
–*Plasmodium ovale* is responsible for ovale and tertian malaria.

History reveals that in the past, malaria disease was present in all parts of the world. However, it now persists predominantly in selected geographical areas. We call these areas where they are present all year round as malaria endemic areas. The regions in the world where malaria is endemic is shown in Fig.4-1.

● Malaria endemic regions

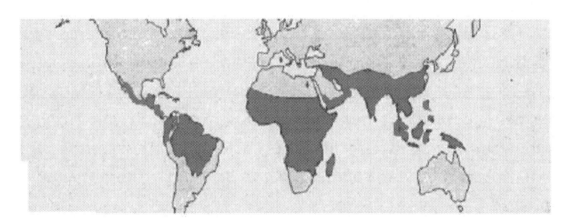

Fig. 4-1: Map of the world showing areas where malaria is endemic (courtesy CDC, Atlanta).

This does not mean that malaria cannot be found in the other parts of the world. American Public Health Authorities report 1200 cases of malaria disease in the United States of America every year. These American reports also indicate that the main source of these cases is travelers arriving in the United States from malaria endemic regions. Infected mosquitoes are also transported into the US by incoming aircraft and ships from malaria endemic regions. Constant surveillance is maintained in regions where malaria has been eradicated as there are still competent mosquito vectors found in these regions capable of transmitting malaria from infected persons to others and start a malaria re-introduction cycle.

It should be remembered that temperature and rainfall are critical to the development and survival of malaria. For example, the Plasmodium parasite cannot complete its cycle inside the Anopheles mosquito at a temperature below 20°C and therefore cannot be a source of infection.

Plasmodium falciparum

The *Plasmodium falciparum* parasite is the most dangerous and the one that kills the most people. The malaria that it causes is called falciparum malaria or malignant malaria. This type of malaria is the most dangerous because it can kill very rapidly. In Africa where it is prevalent, its host mosquito carriers are the *Anopheles gambiae* and the *Anopheles funestus*.

The *Plasmodium falciparum* parasite is found mostly in Africa, Haiti and New Guinea.

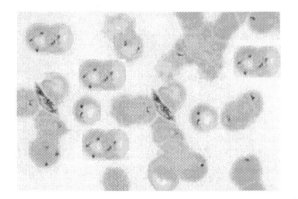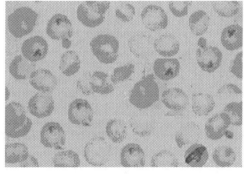

Fig. 4-2: (left) Stained red blood cells infected with falciparum malaria (left) and with quartan malaria (right). Faciparum infection shows many 'ring form' stage cells and banana shaped gametocytes. Quartan infection shows trophozoites as a band inside the non-swelling cells.

Plasmodium malariae

The *Plasmodium malariae* parasite is responsible for quartan malaria. Quartan malaria is characterized by the onset of fever symptoms, including shivering, cold and headache every 72 hours. This parasite is found mostly in Tropical and Sub-tropical Africa.

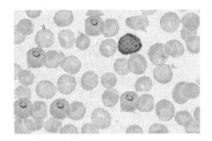 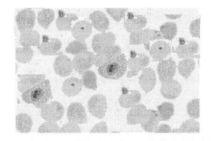

Fig. 4-3: Stained red blood cells infected with tertian malaria (left) and with ovale infection (right). Note the swollen cells and the large stained gametocyte in vivax infections (left) and the oval shaped red blood cells with 'ring form stage' and oval shapes in ovale infections (right)
courtesy CDC

Plasmodium vivax

The *Plasmodium vivax* parasite is responsible for tertian malaria. Another parasite *Plasmodium ovale* is also responsible for tertian malaria. Tertian malaria is characterized by the onset of fever symptoms including, shivering, cold and headache every 48 hours or every other day. *Plasmodium vivax* parasite is mostly found in India, Asia, Oceania as well as South and Central America.

Plasmodium ovale

The *Plasmodium ovale* parasite is responsible for ovale malaria. In ovale malaria, the infected red blood cells often acquire an oval shape. *Plasmodium ovale* is also responsible for tertian malaria. The tertian malaria type is usually mild in form and may be responsible for only a few attacks. Ovale malaria can often be treated with chloroquine. The parasite is mostly found in Africa and Southern India.

In most areas, malaria tests depend on the presence of antigens detected by pricking the finger of the patient. The sensitivity observed with these finger-pricking tests are said to be equivalent to that obtained from a microscopic examination of the patient's blood specimen.

Once a person is exposed to malaria, the patient develops antibodies in the blood. However, the presence of antibodies does not indicate the time of infection or whether the patient still has infection.

HOW THIS PARASITE IS INTRODUCED INTO HUMANS

In 1880, a French Army Doctor, Charles Laveran, found malaria parasites in the red blood cell of his patients. However, it was an Indian born British scientist called Ronald Ross who described the developing parasites in the intestines of mosquitoes and proved that mosquitoes played a vital role in the malaria disease process. Ronald Ross went on to demonstrate the life cycle of the plasmodium parasite in mosquitoes. Today, we know that mosquitoes play a carrier role in the infection process and the spread of the disease.

The life cycle of the parasite ......and its transmission in humans

The life cycle of the Plasmodium parasite is divided into three distinct stages. These are the:

1. human liver stage: this is the period when the parasite is introduced into the human host, develops in the liver and is released into the blood stream.   It is also called the *exo-erythrocytic stage.*

2. red blood stage: this is the period when the parasite enters the red blood cell, develops within it and destroys it. This stage is also called the *erythrocytic stage.*

3. mosquito stage: this is the period when the parasite develops within the mosquito. This stage is also called the *sporogonic stage.*

For convenience and easier comprehension however, we shall discuss these three stages under six periods. These are:

1. the period of plasmodium parasite introduction into human blood

2. the period where the parasite travels to the human liver, enters and multiplies within

3. the period when the parasites leave the human liver to re-enter the blood stream

4. the periods of parasite release in large numbers into the blood stream

5. the period of sexual development of the parasites inside the red blood cell

6. the period of parasite development within the mosquito and its preparation to re-infect   other humans.

 Let us look at how this happens.

Stage 1:   The female mosquito introduces the Plasmodium parasites into human blood.

This is the first stage of the infection process and involves the period when an infected female mosquito sucks blood from a human victim. During this process, the female mosquito injects certain substances into the patient. These substances prevent the victim from feeling pain and the blood from clotting. At the same time, a sizable number of Plasmodium parasites, called *sporozoites*, varying from 5-200, are injected into the human victim's blood. These sporozoites are thin, worm like structures.

As soon as the sporozoites enter the human bloodstream, they find their way directly to the human liver. It takes them only a few minutes to infect the human liver cells.

Stage 2: The sporozoites travel to the human liver and multiply (they change from sporozoites to trophozoites then to merozoites.)

As soon as the sporozoites enter the liver cells, they lose their surface coat (an apical complex) and become *trophozoites*. Inside the liver cell, these trophozoites divide and multiply to become *merozoites*. When these merozoites mature, the liver cells break open and release them into the blood stream. There are usually hundreds of these merozoites inside a liver cell. After release from the liver cells, they do not re-enter the liver cells again. In all respects, they have finished all business with the liver cells. They will not re-infect the liver cells again.

The stage of the plasmodium parasite's life within the liver cell varies from 5-6 days. However, some sporozoites may stay within liver cells for about 2-4 weeks. In some cases, the parasite may stay dormant in the liver cells for a much longer period of time, maybe even for years. During this period, the human host may show no symptoms of the disease.

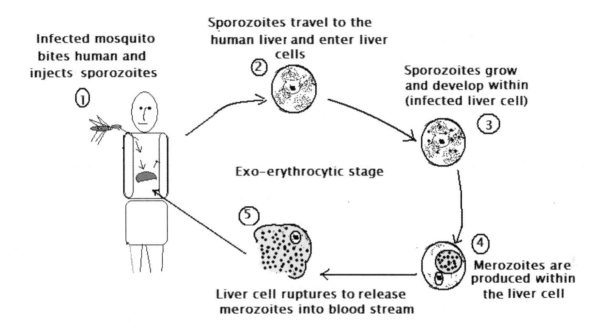

Fig. 4-4: The stages where the parasite enters the liver and develops in the liver cell. This is called the exo-erythrocytic stage (courtesy Dr. Oteng Gyang).

Stage 3: The parasites leave the liver cells and re-enter the blood stream

After these merozoites leave the liver cells and enter the blood stream, they now:

    -penetrate the red blood cells which carry hemoglobin

    -break down hemoglobin which the red blood cells use to carry oxygen and

    -multiply in large numbers inside these red blood cells.

By breaking down hemoglobin, the parasites reduce blood oxygen transport within the human host because the hemoglobin they break down is the human body's main oxygen carrier.

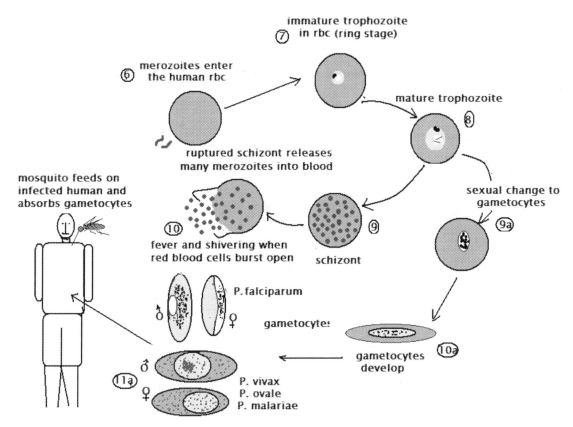

Fig. 4- 5: The stage where the parasite lives and develops in the human red blood cell. This stage is called the erythrocytic stage (courtesy Dr. Oteng Gyang)

This period of merozoite maturation within the blood cell can be divided into three stages. These are:

1. –ring stage

2.–trophozoite stage

3.–schizonts stage

(1) Ring stage: As soon as the merozoites enter the red blood cell, they lose their surface coat (and apical complex – these are called specific invasion organelles) and change into young, round trophozoites. These immature trophozoites constitute a 'ring' stage inside the red blood cell. The ring stage got its name from the fact that when the red blood cell is stained, the immature trophozoites appear in the form of a ring inside the red blood cell.

(2) Trophozoite stage: These young trophozoites grow in size to become large trophozoites.

(3) Schizont stage: These large trophozoites now mature, and each one of them divides further to form 16–18 merozoites within the red blood cell.

These parasites use the hemoglobin of the human victim at this stage for their growth and survival. This process therefore leads to destruction of the human red blood cells resulting in anemia.

Stage 4: Many daughter merozoites are released into the blood stream

More importantly, every forty eight hours, the red blood cells engorged with daughter merozoites rupture and release large numbers of merozoites into the blood stream. These newly released merozoites then re-enter and re-infect other red blood cells and then multiply again within the infected red blood cells.

The simultaneous rupture of large numbers of red blood cells produces chills, shivering, fever, sweating and anemia in the human host. In addition, infected red blood cells travel through the blood stream and enter vital organs like the kidney, heart, brain, liver and other human tissues. When this happens, kidney function is impaired and may lead to kidney failure. The heart starts to overwork due to the reduction in blood supply. Inside the brain, infected, engorged red blood cells obstruct blood vessel channels drastically reducing oxygen supply to the brain leading to the risk of brain oxygen starvation. When the brain is thus starved of oxygen, the process can lead to coma and death. This is cerebral malaria.

Stage 5: Some merozoites change to a sexual stage becoming gametocytes

While in the blood of the human host, some of the merozoites change to a sexual stage, which means some become "males," others become "females." These new sexually transformed parasites are called **gametocytes**. This process of change from a merozoite to a gametocyte takes 10 days. These new sexual parasites now called gametocytes remain within the red blood cells. When a female mosquito sucks blood from this infected human, it takes up some of these newly formed gametocytes. These gametocytes therefore end up inside the intestines of the female mosquito where they undergo the final stage of the transmission cycle, called the **sporogonic** stage.

Stage 6: These gametocytes grow inside the mosquito and become sporozoites again

Inside the mosquito's intestines, the gametocytes undergo further development which changes them back to sporozoites again. This is how it happens.

First, the newly entered gametocytes leave the red blood cell within which they entered the mosquito's gut. The male and the female gametes now undergo different developments. The female gamete just grows, increases in size and becomes spherical. On the other hand, the male gamete divides to form eight cells each with a tail (also called a *flagella).*

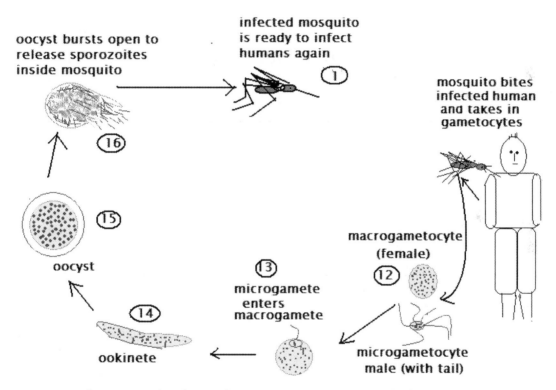

Fig. 4-6: The period when the parasite stays and develops inside the mosquito. This stage is called the sporogonic stage. (courtesy Dr. Oteng Gyang)

The male cell with the flagella then combines with the large spherical female cell to form a *zygote*. This zygote then changes to form an *ookinete*. The ookinete then becomes modified to become an *oocyst*. The oocyst then matures, producing **sporozoites**, which then move into the mosquito's salivary glands. There, they wait to be transmitted to another human host when the mosquito bites another human being and sucks blood from the human host. This process then begins the whole cycle once again.

These changes are presented below:

Male gamete + female gamete --> zygote -->ookinete --> oocyst --> sporozoite

It takes two weeks for gametocyte transformation to sporozoite to be complete inside the mosquito. Therefore it takes a newly infected mosquito two weeks before its newly acquired gametocytes become ready as sporozoites to begin a new transmission and infective cycle again.

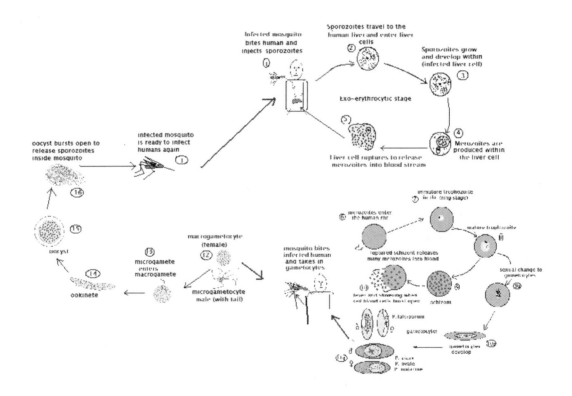

Fig. 4-7: Complete Life cycle of Plasmodium, the malaria parasite (courtesy Dr. Oteng Gyang)

DIAGNOSING MALARIA....

Malaria is diagnosed by its symptoms. It is confirmed by microscopic examination of a blood sample taken from the patient. Such a blood sample will usually show different parasites at different stages of development. It is best to take the blood sample from an infected patient when the patient has an increasing temperature. If tests on three consecutive days do not show the presence of parasites, it can be said that the patient does not have malaria.

TREATMENT OF MALARIA

Modern science-based medicine has documented the use of two main plants in the treatment of malaria. These are the:

1. Cinchona tree from South America, from whose bark **quinine** is obtained.

2. Qinghao tree (Artemisia annua L) from China, and from which **artemisinin** is obtained.

Unknown and unsung heroes in the fight against malaria are a variety of little known African medicinal plants that African herbalists and traditional doctors have used for the treatment of malaria since the beginning of time. We shall discuss these plants when we have looked at the products from the cinchona and qinghao trees.

CINCHONA: THE QUININE PLANT

Quinine is obtained from the bark of the Cinchona tree and is reported to have been used to treat malaria since the seventeenth century. It was named Cinchona by Linnaeus in 1742. Quinine was isolated from its bark by French scientists in 1820 and used to treat intermittent fever.

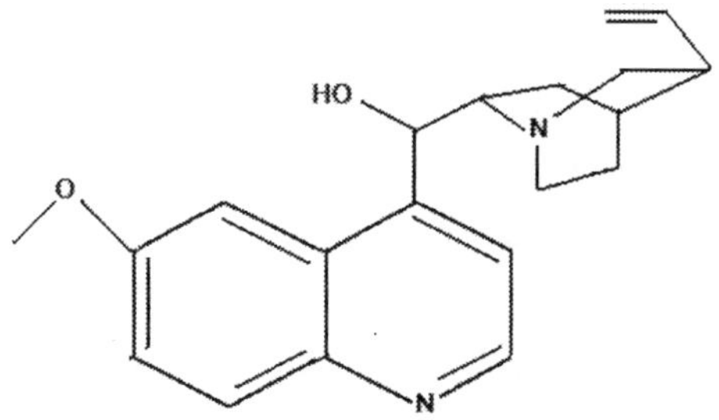

Quinine

(R)-(6-methoxyquinolin-4-yl)(2S,4S,8R)-8- vinylquinuclidin-2-yl)methanol

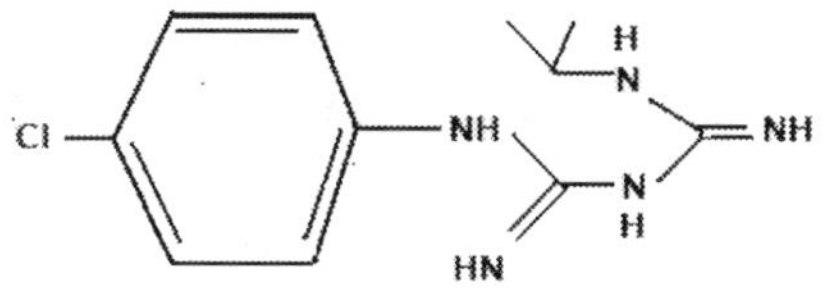

Proguanil

1-(4-chlorophenyl)-2-

(N'-propan-2- ylcarbamimidoyl)quanidine

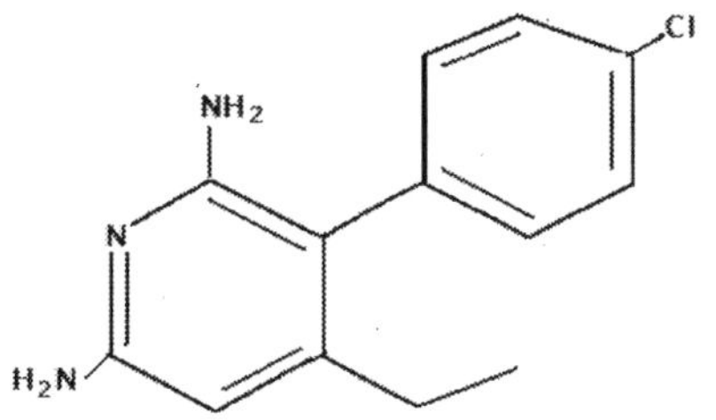

Pyrimethamine

5-(4-chlorophenyl)-6-ethyl-2,4 pyrimidinediamine

Fig. 5-1: Chemical structures of Quinine, Proguanil and Pyrimethamine

Since then, and until quite recently, quinine and quinine derivatives have continued to be the first line of defense against malaria infections. In recent times however, the malaria parasites have shown strong resistance to most of these quinine derivatives, thus reducing their efficacy. The deadly nature of the malaria disease coupled with the urgent need to find acceptable remedies have intensified the scientific quest for more effective drugs.

The following is the list of substances introduced in the fight against malaria and the period plasmodium parasite resistance was observed.

Substance	Year introduced	First case of resistance noted
Quinine	1632	1910
Chloroquine	1945	1957
Proguanil	1948	1949
Sulfadoxine-Pyrimethamine	1967	1967
Mefloquine	1977	1982
Atovaquone	1996	1996

Table 5-1: Malaria treatment drugs and the year plasmodium resistance to them was first noted (source: Global defence against the infectious disease threat, World Health Organization, 2003)

...then came chloroquine

The need to enhance the effectiveness of quinine led scientists to search for synthetic versions of quinine. In 1934, German scientists synthesized 2 new compounds closely related to the chemical structure of quinine. These were **chloroquine** (resochin) and **3-methyl-chloroquine** (sontochin). These compounds constituted a new classs of anti-malaria drugs called the **4-amino-quinolines**.

After the Second World War, chloroquine was produced in the USA. Combined with DDT, a powerful insecticide, these two became the foot soldiers in a world wide program to eradicate malaria. However, the malaria causing parasite, *Plasmodium falciparum* soon developed resistance to chloroquine in different parts of the world. This happened simultaneously in Thai-Cambodia in 1957, Venezuela in 1960, Papua New Guinea in the mid 1970s, Kenya, Tanzania around the late 1970s and Sudan, Uganda, Zambia as well as Malawi around 1983.

...so sulfadoxine and pyrimethamine came to the rescue

During the Second World War, another anti-malarial drug called proguanil (a pyrimidine derivative) was discovered. This drug was successfully used to treat malaria. From it was derived a drug called pyrimethamine.

However, a year later, the malaria parasite developed resistance to proguanil. Not too soon after, parasite resistance to pyrimethamine was also recorded. Subsequently, these two drugs were combined with sulfa based compounds like sulfones and sulfonamides in an effort to increase efficacy and forestall the development of drug resistance by the parasite.

However, it was only a question of time. By 1953, resistant organisms had been discovered in Tanzania. A combined drug of Sulfadoxine/ Pyrimethamine called SP, was released in Thailand in 1967. In the same year, resistant parasites were found. Subsequently, SP– parasite resistant strains spread very fast, not only in Thailand but also into the far corners of Southeast Asia. By the middle of the 1990's resistance to SP had spread to many parts of Africa and the drug had become useless in the fight against malaria.

...then came mefloquine to the rescue

The United States Army Medical Research and Development Command, the World Health Organization and Hoffman La Roche, a European Pharmaceutical company then collaborated in developing another anti-malarial drug called **mefloquine**. It was a drug that was initially meant to prevent malaria. It proved its worth. It was successfully used as a prophylactic against malaria.

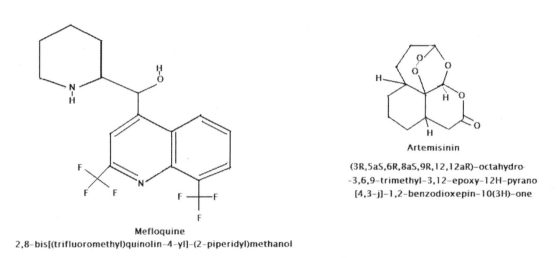

Mefloquine
2,8-bis[(trifluoromethyl)quinolin-4-yl]-(2-piperidyl)methanol

Artemisinin
(3R,5aS,6R,8aS,9R,12,12aR)-octahydro-3,6,9-trimethyl-3,12-epoxy-12H-pyrano[4,3-j]-1,2-benzodioxepin-10(3H)-one

Fig. 5-2: Chemical structures of Mefloquine and Artemisinin

Fortunately, in 1974, it was also found to be effective in malaria treatment and was therefore used to this effect. Mefloquine chalked some success in the fight against malaria on these two fronts: as a prophylactic and as a treatment drug. However, by 1985, like all the others which had come before it, mefloquine was found to have lost its effectiveness in the fight against malaria treatment in several parts of Asia. In short, the malaria parasite had developed resistance to it.

ARTEMISIA ANNUA L. : the artemisinin plant

In 1972, Chinese scientists isolated a new drug from an Asian shrub called Chinese wormwood or *Artemisia annua L.* Hitherto, Chinese traditional herbalists had used this plant for well over 2000 years to treat malaria and other diseases. This new isolate was called artemisinin. In 1979, after seven years of laboratory research, human scientific testing of artemisinin as a treatment drug for malaria was began. Artemisinin proved to be effective in the treatment of malaria.

Subsequent research aimed at the development and improved methods of artemisinin isolation has led to the development of artemisinin related compounds. Prominent among these are the artemether group drugs which are now being used to treat drug resistant forms of malaria.

Research results have proved that Artemisinin and its derivatives enable:

-significant reduction in the plasmodium parasite's biomass in the infected patient

-significant reduction in numbers of *P. falciparum* multi-drug resistant strains

-large reduction in gametocyte numbers and

-rapid resolution of patient symptoms.

Although artemisinin is effective, it has one major drawback. It exhibits a very short half-life and therefore requires several dose regimens at relatively short intervals to enable a complete cure. It is also for this reason that it cannot be used as a stand alone drug.

Currently, therefore, artemisinin in combination with other anti-malarials is the drug of choice in the treatment of malaria. Due to its importance, and the need to forestall the possibility of parasite resistance, the WHO has recommended that artemisinin and its derivates should not be used as stand alone drugs, but must be used in combination with other anti-malarials in any malaria treatment protocol.

The advantages of using artemisinin in combination with other drugs (called Artemisinin combined therapy or ACT) in malaria therapy are as follows:

-prolongation of time that the drug is present and effective in the patient before being broken down and excreted

-reduction of treatment period

-reduction of possible resistance development to artemisinin

-increase in treatment efficacy.

Artemisia annua Plant Cultivation

Artemisia annua L. grows in temperate regions of the world. It grows in the wild in China and Vietnam.

Due to its usefulness as an anti-malarial plant, efforts are being made to produce improved cultivars for commercial propagation. More scientific and agronomic research on new seed developments are underway to find higher artemisinin yielding varieties. Such efforts have already led to the development of varieties that can produce up to 4 tons of dry leaf per hectare with an artemisinin content of about 1.2 percent. More recently, it has been possible to grow some of these varieties in tropical highland areas.

Concurrently, it is reported that commercial plantations are being set up in India, Africa and other parts of Asia in order to meet the increasing need for artemisinin.

Extraction of artemisinin from leaves

Traditional extraction of artemisinin from leaves uses –n–hexane as solvent. N-hexane is relatively cheap and easy to obtain. However it appears to be poisonous and flammable. Therefore, some environmentalists have expressed concerns about its use. As a result, there is new research to find new acceptable solvents. Among the new solvents being proposed are ethanol, hydro–fluorocarbons (HFC), ionic liquids and supercritical carbon dioxide.

After extraction of artesiminin from the leaf source, the product is purified and processed into a wide range of artemisinin derivatives. Some of these derivatives are:
–dihydroartemisinin (DHA)
–Artesunate
–Arteether
–Artemether.

Current recommendations for *Plasmodium falciparum* malaria treatment

Currently, one of these artemisinin derivatives may then be combined with other anti-malarials from the quinine class of compounds, like amodiaquine or piperaquine, to provide an artemisinin-based combination therapy (ACT) product. It is these ACTs that are currently being used in the treatment of malaria.

The following are the recommendations made by the WHO for treatment of uncomplicated malaria:

- artemether–lumefantrine
- artesunate + amodiaquine
- artesunate + mefloquine
- artesunate + sulfadoxine-pyrimethamine.

Other combination drugs proposed by Medicine for Malaria ventures (MMV), a Swiss malaria research corporation include:

* artesunate + chlorproquanil-dapsone
* artesunate + pyronaridine.

However, there are currently no research results on the generalized use of these last two combination drugs in malaria treatment centers and health clinics in Africa.

........treatment of complicated Plasmodium falciparum malaria

For complicated cases of malaria, the WHO recommends the use of artesunate, artemisinin or arthemeter or quinine by intra-muscular, intravenous or rectal routes. In cases of convulsions, pulmonary edema, anemia, low blood sugar, kidney failure and/or coma, additional treatment will be necessary.

........treatment of pregnant women

When women are pregnant, they are treated for malaria in a different way. The WHO recommended treatment for pregnant women depends on the stage of pregnancy and is presented in Table 5-2.

Stage of pregnancy	recommended treatment
1 – 3 months of pregnancy	quinine + clindamycin
4 - 9 months of pregnancy	artesunate +clindamycin or
	quinine + clindamycin or
	quinine + the type of ACT which is effective in the geographical area

Table 5-2: WHO recommendations for the treatment of malaria infected pregnant women.

............treatment of infections with Plasmodium vivax or Plasmodium ovale

Human infections with *Plasmodium vivax and/or Plasmodium ovale* result in these parasites finding refuge in both the human liver and in red blood cells for long periods of time. In most cases, these parasites continue to stay in the human victim's liver and red blood cells long after the patient has undergone successful treatment of the primary infection. Plasmodium parasites that find shelter in the human victim's liver and red blood cells are often released at a later time and cause secondary malaria infections. Therefore, it is very essential to rid these two areas of the body free from the parasites to avoid a relapse of the infection. To this effect, two drugs are used in combination. The drug primaquine targets the liver parasites and kills those parasites which find refuge in it. The second drug, amodiaquine targets those *Plasmodium ovale* and *Plasmodium vivax* parasites which remain in the red blood cells. Therefore, it is essential to ensure that patients who have suffered primary malaria infections from *Plasmodium ovale* and *Plasmodium vivax* undergo a secondary treatment after the primary infectious treatment is over, in order to ensure a complete cure.

Therefore the recommended treatment for *P ovale and P vivax* is summarized as follows

*primaquine + chloroquine or

*amodiaquine + primaquine for chloroquine resistant *Plasmodium vivax* strains.

It is unusual to find very severe cases of *P. ovale or P. vivax* malaria. However, in cases they are discovered, the WHO recommends the same treatment protocol as for severe *P. falciparum*.

.....treatment of malaria infections with Plasmodium malariae

Chloroquine is the WHO recommended drug of choice for the treatment of malaria infections by *Plasmodium malariae*.

...treatment of malaria caused by mixed parasites/ mixed malaria infections

In many countries, malaria infections are mixed and result from infections with several parasites. Such is the case in Thailand where about a third of patients with acute *Plasmodium falciparum* infections are observed to be infected with *Plasmodium vivax* as well. Artemisinin combined therapy are the drugs of choice for mixed malaria infections with primaquine being recommended additionally for those co-infected with *Plasmodium ovale and Plasmodium vivax*.

OTHER DRUGS

..synthetic drugs

There is some research being done in some private drug manufacturing companies and research institutions with the view to find entirely new synthetic drugs that will replace quinine and artemisinin. Due to the world-wide nature of the malaria problem and the need to coordinate efforts on a global scale, the need for a public-private combined efforts have been suggested. Such initiatives have seen the birth of a malaria research organization like Medicines for Malaria Ventures (MMV) based in Switzerland. This MMV organization's research hopes to develop new anti-malarials that could be used in combination therapies. Efforts are also being made to develop synthetic peroxides that are cheaper, easier to manufacture and are not derived from artemisinin.

.......African drugs...and research into them

Some bottled pharmaceutical liquid products are currently being sold in African pharmacies particularly in Ghana. Such drugs appear to have received marketing and scientific approval by the Ghanaian Standards Board and the Ghanaian Traditional Herbalists Drug Research center at Manpong, Ghana. These endorsements indicate that these preparations do have their usefulness in the national arsenal in the fight against malaria. Unfortunately, little attention is paid to these products by the international research institutions that are currently vying to unearth new drugs to fight this deadly disease.

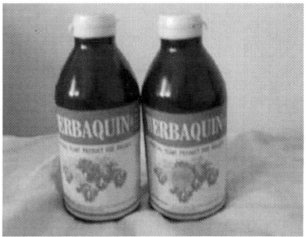

Fig 5-3: African herbal preparation used in the treatment of malaria in Ghana (photo Dr Oteng Gyang)

...diet in the treatment of malaria

Naturopathy suggests that diet plays an important role in the treatment of malaria. Some naturopathy experts suggest that a faulty life style leads to the human system being clogged with systemic refuse and it is on these that the parasites thrive. They suggest that the liberal consumption of meat, canned and denatured foods as well as alcoholic beverages decrease the body's ability to protect itself making it vulnerable to malaria infections. Naturopathy suggests that infected patients should fast on orange juice for a few days depending on the severity of the disease. After fasting for a few days, patients could eat a well balanced diet of natural foods with lots of fresh foods and vegetables. Unfortunately, there are no documented results on the use of this protocol in the effective treatment of malaria.

.......new approaches to finding the silver bullet to kill malaria in Africa

It could be argued that the therapy for an endemic disease is usually found where the disease is endemic. Natural laws would suggest that where an organism is abundant, there will its natural predators also be found. This would suggest that natural predators for the mosquito should be found in Africa. It is also possible that natural therapies for the destruction of the plasmodium parasite could be found amid the millions of plant species that grow wild in Africa. Do African herbalists have knowledge that is being overlooked in this global fight for which the major battleground is Africa? Should humanity take a more critical look at what African herbalists have been using to fight and cure malaria since the beginning of time and help use current technology to refine their efforts?

This is the approach that is being taken by the STOP MALARIA NOW FOUNDATION based in the USA (Atlanta) and Africa (Accra, Ghana). Since there are currently many African research scientists, engineers, it stands to reason that these scientists be mobilized in a collaborative effort with local indigenes to tackle this major problem that affects their lives on a daily basis. This organization seeks to mobilize African human, social, community as well as Africa's indigenous, botanical and scientific resources in a fruitful collaborative effort with the rest of the world in the fight to eradicate malaria as a matter of urgency.

MALARIA PREVENTION DRUGS

Most drugs that have the capacity to treat malaria can also be used in smaller doses to prevent malaria infections. More often, travelers from the Northern hemisphere and other areas where malaria has been eradicated are often advised to take these drugs when visiting malaria-risk countries. Some people living in malaria endemic regions also take some of these drugs on a regular basis to ward off infections. Travelers who visit malaria endemic regions briefly, can significantly reduce their chances of contracting malaria with regular intake of these drugs during their period of stay in these areas and after (for a few months) coupled with the use of insecticide-treated bed nets.

To date, the main drugs used in the prevention of malaria are:
- atovaquone/proguanil
- chloroquine phosphate
- doxycycline
- hydroxychloroquine sulfate
- mefloquine
- primaquine

ATOVAQUONE/PROGUANIL   (Brand name: malarone)

Administration: Oral: 1 adult tablet per day.

An adult tablet is 250mg atovaquone/100mg proguanil.

Children doses depend on the weight of the child.

When taken: The first tablet is taken 1 or 2 days before travel to the malaria endemic region. It should be taken with food or milk at the same time each day.

How often during travel: One tablet every day during the period of stay in the malaria endemic region.

How long after return should the drug be taken: One tablet is taken every day for the next seven days after return from the malaria endemic region.

Side Effects: Most common side effects are stomach pain, vomiting, nausea and headache.

Warning: The following people should not take atovaquone/proguanil:

- -pregnant women
- -women who are breast-feeding babies
- -babies who weigh less than 5 kilograms
- -anyone who is allergic to atovaquone/proguanil.

CHLOROQUINE PHOSPHATE   (Brand names: several; one of them is aralen)

Chloroquine resistance has been observed in many parts of Africa and Asia. It is possible that many other countries have chloroquine resistant parasites too. However, the United States Centers for Disease Control direct that people traveling to Mexico, the Caribbean, certain countries in Central America, the Middle East and Eastern Europe may take chloroquine as their anti-malarial drug.

Administration: Oral dose is 500 mg chloroquine phosphate once a week. Children dose is weight related and is also taken once a week.

When taken: Take the first chloroquine phosphate dose 1 week before you travel. Always take chloroquine after you have eaten, or on a full stomach.

How often during travel period: Take 500 mg of chloroquine phosphate once a week during the period of travel.

How long after return should the drug continue to be taken: Take 500mg chloroquine phosphate once a week for 4 weeks after return from the malaria risk region.

Side Effects: Most common side effects include vomiting, nausea, blurred vision, itching headache and dizziness.

Warning: The following people should not take chloroquine:

-those who are allergic to chloroquine

-those traveling to regions where there are chloroquine-resistant parasites. These regions include many parts of Asia and sub-Saharan Africa.

DOXYCYCLINE (Brand names: several. Doxycycline is a form of tetracycline)

Administration: Oral: the adult dosage is 100mg once a day. The dose for children, over 8 years of age, is also once a day and depends on the weight of the child.

When taken: The first tablet is taken 1 or 2 days before travel to the malaria- risk region.

How often during travel: One tablet every day, at the same time each day, during the period of stay in the malaria-risk area.

How long after return should the drug be taken: One tablet each day for 4 weeks after return from the malaria risk region.

Side Effects: Most common side effects include nausea, stomach pain and sun-sensitivity. Proper dressing with a hat and sun-glasses can alleviate the problem with sun sensitivity. It has been reported that some women on doxycycline develop vaginal yeast infections, leading to malodorous discharge, itching and offensive odors. Such problems may be alleviated with a prescription drug or an over-the-counter anti-yeast medication.

Warning: The following people should not take doxycycline:

-anyone allergic to doxycyclines or tetracyclines

- pregnant women

-children below the age of 8 years

HYDROXYCHLOROQUINE SULFATE (Brand name:Plaquenil)

Hydroxychloroquine sulfate is available as an alternative drug to chloroquine phosphate.

Administration: Oral: 1 adult tablet per week. An adult tablet is 400mg of hydroxychloroquine phosphate. The dose for children depends on the weight of the child and is also taken once a week.

When taken: The first tablet is taken 1 week before travel to the malaria-risk area. The hydroxychloroquine sulfate tablet should be taken after eating. This will help avoid nausea and vomiting.

How often during travel: One tablet every week, on the same day, during whole period of stay in the malaria-risk area.

How long after return should the drug be taken: The same dose should be taken once a week for 4 weeks after return from the malaria-risk region.

Side Effects: Most side effects include nausea, vomiting, headache, dizziness, blurred vision, itching and a bad taste in the mouth.

Warning: The following people should not take hydroxyl-chloroquine sulfate:

   –those who are allergic to hydroxychloroquine

   –those traveling to areas where there are chloroquine resistant malaria parasites. This includes many parts of Asia and sub-Saharan Africa.

MEFLOQUINE   (Brand name: Lariam and many generics)

Administration: Oral: 1 adult tablet per week.

An adult tablet is 250mg of mefloquine. The dose for children depends on the weight of the child and it is taken once a week.

When taken: The first tablet is taken 1 or 2 weeks before travel to the malaria endemic region.

How often during travel: One tablet once a week, on the same day during the whole period of stay in the malaria risk region. Mefloquine should be taken after meals or with a full glass of milk.

How long after return should the drug be taken: Once a week on the same day for 4 weeks after arrival from the malaria-risk region.

Side Effects: Most common side effects include anxiety, vivid dreams, visual disturbances and sleeping difficulties. Others include headache, dizziness and   nausea.

Lesser side effects have been observed with mefloquine levels used to prevent malaria. More frequent side effects are seen with the higher doses used to treat malaria.

Warning: The following people may not take mefloquine:
- those allergic to mefloquine
- those who have cardiac problems such as irregular heartbeats
- those who have a history of seizures
- those with anxiety disorders, schizophrenia
- those with a history of depression or are being treated for depression
- those with a history of psychosis or psychiatric disorders.

PRIMAQUINE

Primaquine may be taken by those traveling to areas where there is Plasmodium vivax (or vivax malaria). However, any such person wishing to take Primaquine should be tested for the presence of an enzyme called Glucose-6-phosphate dehydrogenase (G6PD). Only those with normal levels of G6PD can take Primaquine. Those who are deficient in this enzyme cannot take primaquine. This is is due to the fact that primaquine can cause red blood cells in G6PD deficient people to burst apart, and this may cause death in such persons.

Administration: Oral: An adult should take 2 tablets of 30mg base primaquine once a day. The dose for children depends on the weight of the child and is also taken once a day.

When taken: The first tablet is taken 1 or 2 days before travel to the malaria risk area.

How often during travel: One tablet at the same time each day, every day during the period of stay in the malaria risk area.

How long after return should the drug be taken: One primaquine tablet of (30mg primaquine base) should be taken each day at the same time for 7 days after returning from the malaria-risk area.

Side Effects: The following people should not take primaquine:

–anyone who is allergic to primaquine

–anyone with a G6PD enzyme deficiency

–anyone who has not had a blood test for G6PD deficiency

–pregnant women (the fetus may be G6PD even if the mother's levels have been tested and found to be normal)

–women who are breast feeding, unless the baby has been tested and found to have normal G6PD enzyme levels.

Chapter 6: MALARIA VECTOR REDUCTION BY PHYSICAL METHODS

Prevention is better than cure. If malaria can be prevented and, or adequately controlled, millions of lives will be spared. In addition, countless millions of people will be relieved from the scourge of this terrible affliction that saps human energy, empties human pockets and makes human lives a living hell.

Efforts aimed at malaria prevention and control divide the subject into two areas of responsibility: those of the **individual** and those that fall within the domain of **public health**. For effective mosquito control, each group must completely meet its obligations.

Currently, the work of mosquito prevention and control is approached under a concept called the Integrated Mosquito Management [IMM] strategy. This concept relies on integrating a particular geographical area's social and economic conditions into effective pest management strategies with the view to improving public health, while doing little or no harm to the environment. Playing a prominent role in this approach is **pest source reduction** also called **vector reduction**. This is a multidisciplinary approach which generally includes the following:

     –physical control methods
     –biological control methods
     –chemical control methods.

These approaches are divided into several categories.

Physical control methods

Physical control methods include the following:

-environmental destruction and elimination of mosquito breeding sites

-the use of bed-nets at night to prevent mosquitoes from feeding on humans

-the use of mosquito screens to protect all house entrances

-the use of catch-and-destroy traps

-the use of sound energy to destroy mosquito larvae

Biological control methods

Biological control methods include:

-the use of natural predators to control adult mosquitoes and larvae

-the use of artificially introduced bacteria to kill mosquito larvae

-the development of an effective vaccine

-sterilization of male mosquitoes by ionizing irradiation

Chemical control methods

Chemical control methods comprise:

-the use of insecticides

-the use of larvicides

-the use of skin products that discourage mosquito bites eg DEET

-the use of non-skin contact repellents like mosquito coils, pyrethroids, etc.

An effective IMM strategy would incorporate all these factors as well as the social and economic realities of a particular geographic area.

PHYSICAL CONTROL METHODS

....environmental issues like getting rid of breeding sites and pools of water

As has already been said, a number of environmental issues help perpetuate the progression of malaria. It is widely known that the mosquito carrier requires stagnant water for breeding and survival. Stagnant water breeding sites include open gutters and drains, empty food tins and cans and abandoned tires. Others are dug-out holes in the ground, abandoned swimming pools, barrels and receptacles for collecting and holding water in homes. Natural sites like tree holes and banks of rivers and streams especially where there are growing weeds and water current is slow, also constitute favorable mosquito breeding grounds. The list is long.

For mosquito control methods to be effective, it is imperative to get rid of all such stagnant water which constitutes breeding areas for mosquitoes on a constant basis. The successful attainment of this objective entails regular inspection of all public places and homes by relevant government and private health authorities. Such methods will include draining gutters, disposing of tins, cans, lorry tires and any other unwanted stagnant water containers. Rain water collection and holding containers like barrels and tanks should be covered to prevent entry by breeding mosquitoes. Open drains create standing water in several difficult-to-reach places and provide suitable mosquito breeding grounds. This is the reason why developing countries should abandon the open drain system in favor of covered drains.

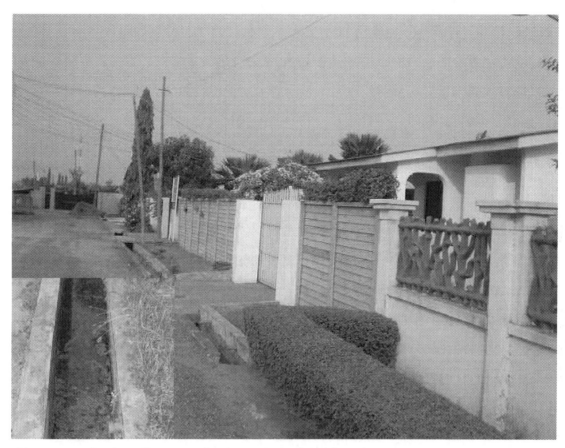

Picture 6-1: Open drains in developing countries, even in middle class suburbs are important breeding grounds for mosquitoes (photo Dr. Oteng Gyang).

In North America, where both public and large private firms work hand in hand to eliminate breeding sites, inspectors often conduct pest source reduction campaigns within selected neighborhoods. These include house to house visits to find, check and reduce the production of mosquitoes and their breeding habitats. Such inspectors educate homeowners on what constitute breeding grounds and breeding habitats and how to destroy them. A similar campaign took place in Ghana and many parts of the world during the period of global malaria eradication program in the nineteen sixties. The same can be done in all parts of the world where malaria exists.

..... the use of bed nets/mosquito nets

Bed nets also called mosquito nets have been used for a long time in malaria endemic areas as a physical barrier between humans and mosquitoes. These nets are often used at night during sleep. Bed nets often consist of a rectangular shaped nylon, polyester or cotton net sewed to fit over a bed. It is normally erected over a bed at night to keep mosquitoes out.

In the past, most bed-net users employed non-insecticide treated bed-nets. These bed-nets were not very efficient because mosquitoes settled on the bed nets and waited for the sleeper's body to roll to a side of the bed where the mosquitoes could have access to the sleeper's skin and feed. The recent introduction of insecticide treated nets has eliminated this problem mainly because insecticide-treated nets kill mosquitoes which settle on them. Insecticide treated nets are therefore an advantage over non-treated nets. It is to this end that the WHO has issued recommendations favoring the use of insecticide treated nets over their non-treated counterparts.

The WHO has also issued recommendations on the types of insecticides to be used in treating bed-nets and the dosages to be employed (Table 6-1). One of such chemical insecticides widely employed to treat bed nets is permethrin. Mosquito-nets that are treated with permethrin retain their effectiveness even after repeated washing. The effectiveness of permethrin treated bed-nets includes prevention and killing of undesirable insects, mostly mosquitoes. To make it easier to use, these formulations are often prepared in dosages and specific easy-to-understand instructions given on what amount of chemical is needed to soak the net and for what period of time.

In 2006, the then President of the United States, George W. Bush began a special United States Presidential Malaria Initiative (PMI) to combat malaria. He called for a 1.2 billion fund to combat malaria morbidity and mortality in 15 African countries (Angola, Tanzania, Uganda, Malawi, Mozambique, Ghana, Senegal, Kenya, Liberia, Zambia, Madagascar, Benin, Rwanda, Mali and Ethiopia). Public and private sector partnerships were encouraged to work together to overcome this scourge.

Later that year, the PMI working with the Global Fund is said to have distributed some 230 000 insecticide treated nets to the people of Zanzibar. As a result Zanzibar, an island off the coast of East Africa, reported a significant reduction in malaria cases and quick recovery times for patients receiving treatment. Significant decreases in malaria cases were also recorded for Pemba Island also off the coast of Tanzania in East Africa (87% reduction in malaria infections from January 2006 to September 2006 as compared to the same period in 2005).

Insecticide	Formulation	Dosage (mg) active ingredient / m^2 of netting
Alpha-cypermetrin	SC 10%	20-40
Cyfluthrin	EW 5%	50
Deltamethrin	SC 1% and WT 25%	15-25
Etofenprox	EW 10%	200
Lambda-cyhalothrin	CS 2.5%	10-15
Permethrin	EC 10%	200-500

EC : emulsifiable concentrate
EW: emulsion, oil in water
CS: capsule suspension
SC: suspension concentrate
WT: water dispersible tablet

Table 6-1: World Health Organization (WHO) recommended insecticides for the treatment of mosquito nets destined to be used for malaria vector control (WHO homepage. www. WHO.int/whopes/en/.

Research by UNICEF and medical research data from Ghana and Kenya indicate that the use of these bed nets reduce malaria infections by 20% in endemic areas and that child deaths may be lessened by up to 30% in these areas.

....the use of mosquito screens on house entrances

Mosquito screens are very fine, inexpensive, plastic netting that is spread over and fixed on windows, doors and entrances to dwelling places to prevent physical entry by mosquitoes and other insects.

Research has shown that some malaria borne mosquito species enter dwelling places, lurk indoors and feed on their human victims. It is only when they are well fed with human blood that these mosquitoes leave these human dwellings to find breeding sites where they lay their eggs. As soon as their eggs are laid outdoors, they return indoors to the human dwelling places to feed again. Therefore, mosquito bed nets may protect people when they sleep, but they offer little by way of protection to those people who watch television, play or stay with other family members in their living rooms, verandahs or bedrooms at dusk or during the night.

An effective way to protect humans would be to prevent mosquito access to human dwelling places. This would mean preventing mosquitoes from gaining physical entry into dwelling places. It is to this end that the use of mosquito netting on doors, windows and all entrances to a dwelling place is useful. Today, mosquito screens are used in several homes in Africa, Asia and the Americas. In such places, they provide an effective physical barrier to mosquito entry into human homes.

.......the use of catch-and-destroy traps

Catch and destroy traps are devices that attract, capture and destroy adult female mosquitoes. They mimic human color, movement, body heat and scent as well as other human chemical emanations with the view to ensnaring female mosquitoes looking for a human blood feed.

For catch and destroy traps to be effective, two important conditions must be met. The first is to lure the mosquito to a location from where it cannot escape. The second is to destroy it. Methods used to lure the mosquito include the use of mosquito attractants like light, human body scent as well as movement and heat. Once it has been caught, the insect is destroyed by starvation and dehydration.

Catch and destroy traps vary widely in their construction, effectiveness and price. Some are simple to make and of low-cost while others are quite sophisticated and rather expensive. Since these catch and destroy traps emphasize different criteria for luring and catching mosquitoes, it is possible that they may vary in their capacity to lure and capture different species of mosquitoes too. Research has indicated that this could be so. Indeed, some traps show a greater tendency to catch certain species of mosquitoes and appear to be indifferent to other species. More research is definitely needed in this area. Nevertheless, it is highly possible that catch and destroy traps could well play an important role in the complete eradication of adult mosquitoes. In view of this, some explanation will be given on the idea behind the function of these traps.

-mosquito attractants: chemical

Mosquitoes are drawn to human prey by **chemical** and **non-chemical attractants**. Chemical attractants include all chemical substances that emanate from humans. In human breath alone, there are over a hundred of these chemical substances. However, extensive scientific research shows that only two of these chemicals attract mosquitoes to a very significant degree. These are **carbon dioxide** and **octenol**. Non chemical attractants include heat, light, scent, color, shape and motion of human bodies. Catch and destroy traps use a combination of these mosquito attractants to capture these deadly insects.

–carbon dioxide

Human beings inhale oxygen and exhale carbon dioxide. Mosquitoes follow the smell of carbon dioxide to detect the presence of human beings to feed on them. Scientific research shows that carbon dioxide can attract mosquitoes from a distance of up to 36 meters (120 feet). Carbon dioxide is therefore an important ingredient in the construction of mosquito catch-and-destroy traps.

–octenol

Octenol (1-octen-3-ol) is a powerful mosquito attractant found in very small quantities in human breath. Like carbon dioxide, mosquitoes can detect its presence in air from a distance of up to 36 meters (120 feet). It therefore constitutes one of the important ingredients in the construction of mosquito traps.

<u>–mosquito attractants: non chemical</u>

During the night, mosquitoes additionally use light, human scent and motion to detect their human prey. Light and motion are therefore called non-chemical attractants.

–long range attractants and short range attractants

Mosquitoes use some of these attractants to detect and follow human beings from long distances. These include light, human scent, motion, carbon dioxide and octenol. These are therefore called **long range attractants**.

Other mosquito attractants are body heat, moisture and lactic acid. Most mosquitoes cannot detect the presence of human body heat, moisture and lactic acid from afar. These three elements therefore serve to direct the mosquito to its target at close range. Body heat, moisture and lactic acid are therefore called **terminal attractants or short range attractants**.

Mosquito catch–and–destroy traps employ both short range and long range attractants to lure and capture female mosquitoes.

Catch–and–destroy methods vary from simple to very sophisticated ones.

A very simple trap for capturing mosquitoes was developed by a class of young children in Taiwan. This involves the use of a waste plastic bottle, cut in half with the top inverted over the base. When a sugary liquid with yeast is poured into the base–half, carbon dioxide is emitted and acts as an attractant for mosquitoes. A modified version of this uses a gourd–calabash that is grown in every village in Africa in lieu of a waste plastic bottle. This modified version, called the **calabash–trap**, was developed by the STOP MALARIA NOW FOUNDATION based in the USA and Africa. The procedure for manufacture of these simple traps is detailed in Fig. 6-1 to 6-8 and can be easily produced at very low cost in every village in Africa.

Procedures for the manufacture of very simple catch-and-destroy traps

The procedures for the manufacture of these simple mosquito traps involve the use of very rudimentary materials that can be easily obtained in every village in Africa and Asia, no matter how remote or how poor its inhabitants are.

Equipment needed

The equipment consists of:

-2000 ml container (an empty plastic bottle or a calabash gourd will do very well)

-50 gram of sugar (brown sugar is good)

-1 gram of Baker's yeast

-a knife

-a black plastic material (black paper will do very well) Step 1:

(A) Cut the plastic bottle in two (B) Cut the calabash gourd in two.

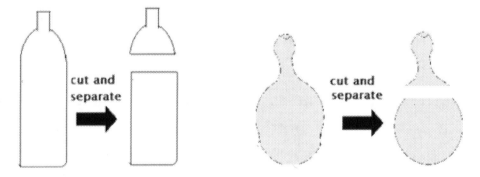

Fig. 6-1: The top end of the plastic bottle or gourd is cut into two and separated.

Step 2: Warm 200 ml (a cup) of water and then add 50 gram of sugar. Stir until it dissolves to produce a sugar solution or syrup. Allow the syrup to cool until about 40° centigrade. [If you have no thermometer, let syrup cool until a drop on the inside of your wrist is not painful].

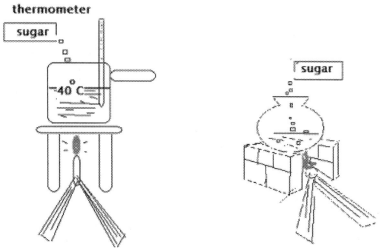

Fig. 6-2: A sugar solution is prepared by dissolving the sugar in warming water.

Step 3: Pour the water with the sugar into the bottom part of the large container (plastic bottle or the calabash gourd.

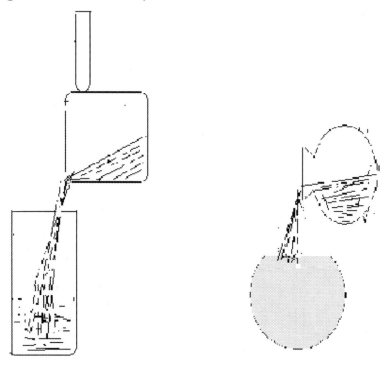

Fig. 6-3: The sugar mixture is poured into the bottom half of the plastic container or into the bottom half of the gourd

Step 4: Sprinkle the yeast on top of the sugary liquid in the plastic bottle or in the calabash. Do not mix the yeast with the sugary mixture.

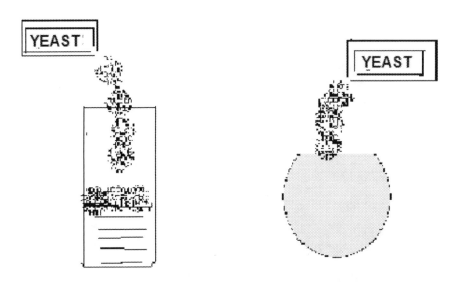

Fig. 6-4: The yeast is sprinkled on top of the sugary mixture in the plastic container or of the gourd.

Step 5: Invert the top of the plastic bottle on the larger plastic container, or the top half of the gourd on top of the bottom half.

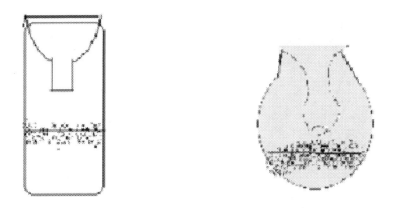

Fig. 6-5: The upper half of the container is inverted on top of the bottom half.

Step 6: Wrap the black plastic material around the plastic bottle. Wrap a strip of black plastic around the top of the gourd firmly to prevent the escape of gas.

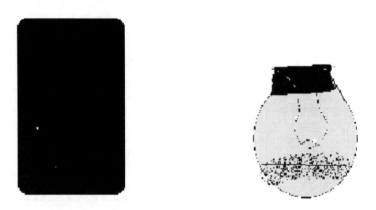

Fig. 6-6: The plastic container is completely wrapped with black plastic. the top of the gourd is wrapped to prevent the entry of air and undesirable objects.

Step 7: Put the wrapped material it in a dark corner of the house outside or inside.

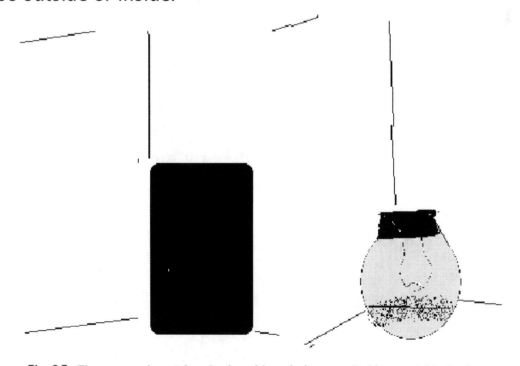

Fig. 6-7: The wrapped container is placed in a dark corner inside or outside the house.

Step 8: Empty the contents every two weeks and change the solution. You may let the children keep count of how many mosquitoes are caught at the end of each 2 week period.

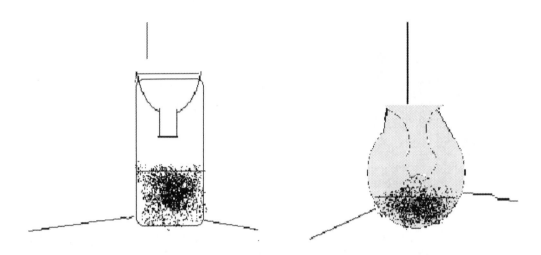

Fig6-8: The containers are inspected every two weeks, emptied and the solution replaced.

....some sophisticated catch-and-destroy traps

More elaborate traps use a combination of attractants to lure the mosquitoes into sophisticated catch-and-destroy traps. These traps and mosquito killing systems operate on the same principle of lure, catch and destroy. Their differences lie in the number of combined attractants employed and the amount of user attention needed for operation. When more attractants are employed in combination with complex electronic gadgetry, less user supervision is required. On the contrary, sophistication and prices go up.

Therefore, the more sophisticated traps use a combination of light, heat, octenol, carbon dioxide attractants and computer chips with electronic circuitry to control automatic performance. In spite of this, the basic unit of these

more complex traps appears to be similar. Most of them have the following:
-a bottle of propane gas which slowly burns propane to produce carbon dioxide gas,   moisture and heat
- an octenol attractant which is slowly heated to evaporate
-ultra-violet light produced by light emitting diodes
-a power source for electric current
- a trap from where the lured mosquito cannot escape and
-a mosquito catch tray

The unit may also have the following:
-a support and stand on which the catch tray is held
-a plastic propane regulator and hose for proper connection to the gas tank
- a fan to blow and disseminate the carbon dioxide and octenol attractants.
 -a vacuum suction action that draws the mosquitoes into a trap where they dehydrate and die
It is also necessary to place the unit in a special location, depending on wind direction in order to maximize mosquito catch.

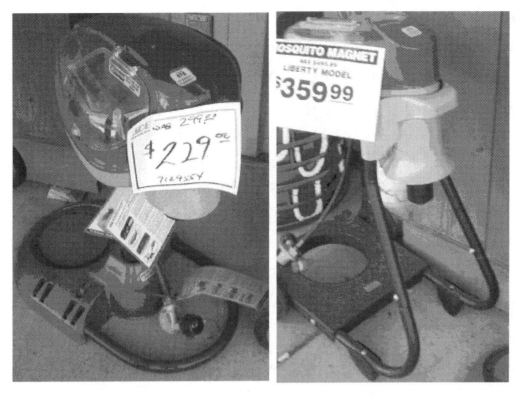

Fig 6-9: Some commercial mosquito catch
and destroy traps (photo: Dr. Oteng Gyang)

Using sound waves to destroy larvae

Some physical control methods aim at the destruction of mosquitoes during their developmental stage. Such methods destroy the adult mosquito, its eggs, larvae and pupae. Prominent among these are those that aim at larva control and destruction. These are called larvicides.

A recent method that has been added to the arsenal of larvae control is an acoustic larva killing system. The idea behind this method came from the high school Science Fair project of Michael Nyberg, a New York state resident and led to the development of an instrument called '**larvasonic.**'

The basic idea behind 'larvasonic' is simple. Mosquito larvae have internal air bladders which they use to breathe. When sound waves are sent through a pool of water containing these larvae, the sound waves make their air bladders vibrate tremendously leading to tissue rupture and death of the larvae.

The first type of 'larvasonic' resembled a small gadget which could be activated by a button and then dropped into a pool of water. Trials in stagnant water containing mosquito larvae showed that any larvae within 3 feet would then die after barely three seconds after activation. Twenty four hours later, those larvae within a five feet radius would also die. Commercial variations of the 'larvasonic' are being marketed. Currently, these include custom tailored installations for industry and wide open spaces.

Chapter 7: MALARIA VECTOR REDUCTION BY BIOLOGICAL AND CHEMICAL METHODS

The subject of biological and chemical control methods has already been introduced in an earlier chapter. The details of these are as follows:

Biological control methods
Biological control methods include:

- the use of natural predators to control adult mosquitoes and larvae
- the use of artificially introduced bacteria to kill mosquito larvae
- the development of an effective vaccine
- sterilization of male mosquitoes by ionizing irradiation

Chemical control methods
Chemical control methods comprise:

- the use of insecticides
- the use of larvicides
- the use of skin products that discourage mosquito bites eg DEET
- the use of non-skin contact repellents like mosquito coils, pyrethroids, etc.

BIOLOGICAL CONTROL METHODS
...the use of natural predators to control adult and larvae

In any ecosystem, any given organism has natural enemies. This is no different for the mosquito. Biological control methods seek to enhance the influence and development of the natural enemies of the mosquito and/or to introduce new predators where they are inefficient, insufficient or absent. Natural predators of the adult mosquito include microorganisms, fish, birds, bats and dragonflies. Research has shown that some types of bacteria are particularly good at destroying growing mosquito larvae. These bacteria are called larvicides. Currently, larvicides offer one of the greatest hopes for malaria control and eradication.

....Bacillus thuringensis and Bacillus sphaericus sp.

Some species of bacteria attack and destroy insects providing an efficient means of biological control. By far, the most successful and the most widely used bacteria are *Bacillus thuringensis israelensis* (Bti) and *Bacillus sphaericus* (Bsh). These bacteria are produced commercially and used in formulations that are safe and easy to apply.

Bti and Bsh are natural soil bacteria that have been developed as larvicides to control the larva stage of mosquitoes. Being bacilli, these two bacteria can produce spores that can be harvested and mixed with inert material to produce a concentrate of easily dispersible material. This dispersible material is then spread on the surfaces of lakes, ponds and stagnant waters. When the larvae ingest the concentrate, the bacteria spores in the concentrate grow and reproduce inside the larvae, where they synthesize crystalline toxins. These crystalline toxins paralyze the digestive tract of the larvae making feeding impossible. Death then follows within 1 to 5 days depending on the type of mosquito.

A typical Bti product would contain 0.8% of bacteria concentrate and about 98.2 of an inert material. Commercial Bti is available in liquid, granular and time-release formulations. Commercial *Bacillus sphaericus* preparations (*VectoLex CG*) have been reported to have a longer residual effect than *Bacillus thuringensis israelensis* preparations (*VectoBac)* and therefore may provide a more extended period of larvae control in a habitat.

Commercial types of Bti come in two forms: **mosquito bits and mosquito briquets.** Manufacturers allege that the Bti mosquito bits can keep a pond free of mosquito larvae for 7 days. Bti may also be used to control the larvae of the black fly and the gnat.

Bacteria insecticide formulations are generally insect specific. Therefore, insecticide formulations that are used to control one type of insect larva may not have any effect on other insect species. Many insecticide formulations that can control various agricultural pests are now commercially available.

Fish in ponds

Some species of fish like to feed on mosquito larvae. The mosquito fish, *Gambusia affinis* is one of such natural predators. When this mosquito fish is introduced into ponds, it feeds on the mosquito larvae, reducing their populations and therefore constitutes some form of biological mosquito control. Whether the presence of the mosquito fish is sufficient by itself to control mosquito populations adequately for long periods of time is an open question. In addition, many ponds and water holding areas may not hold sufficient water, all year round to enable the survival of the mosquito fish. It should be remembered that, in several tropical countries, many streams and ponds dry out during the dry season. The drying out of a stream or pond would put the survival of the fish at stake. This could jeopardize the sustainable nature of a mosquito control project. However, the breeding and introduction of these fishes into pools, streams, drainage canals and gutters with sufficient water for long periods of the year could contribute an additional arsenal in the fight to reduce mosquito populations. Furthermore, in tropical nations, such fish could also provide an important source of additional income as well as a good source of protein for local people.

Birds, Bats, Dragonflies, and Frogs that feed on mosquitoes

Some birds like purple martins have been introduced into mosquito habitats to help control mosquito populations. Other predators like bats, dragonflies and frogs have also been used but reports about significant successes have been anecdotal and few.

Spiders

Some spiders in East Africa eat the Anopheles mosquitoes that cause malaria. Researchers Jackson and Nelson from New Zealand have reported that a spider, *(Evarcha culicivora)* found near Lake Victoria, East Africa singles out the malaria causing female Anopheles mosquito for food,. These 5mm long spiders with very keen eyesight have been observed to jump about 20 cm to catch and feed on these mosquitoes. Such spiders could provide some amount of control for mosquitoes that rest indoors or outdoors on walls of human dwelling places.

.....insect growth regulator products (s-methoprene)

Methoprene is a synthetic insect growth regulator hormone which interferes with mosquito larvae development. It is approved in many parts of the world for the killing and destruction of larvae. It is very effective against the *Culex spp* of mosquitoes but shows very low toxicity towards non-target species.

Commercial preparations are available as methoprene pellets or briquets (Altosid, (registered trade name). Reports from Canada indicate that methoprene is more effective than *Bacillus thuringensis israelensis* or *Bacillus sphaericus* in the control of mosquito larvae. Larvaciding treatments of mosquito breeding sites in Canada indicate that methoprene can keep water basins 100% free of mosquito larvae for up to 21 days.

.........the development of an effective vaccine

The history of using mild forms of a disease to infect people in order to protect them against more deadly versions of the same disease have been recorded in China, India and Turkey since 200 BCE. However, it was not until the much publicized smallpox experimental observations of the British Surgeon, Edward Jenner, in 1796 did the use of vaccines become largely acceptable. Ever since, vaccines have played an important role in disease control and eradication in many countries of the modern world. It is therefore normal to resort to vaccine research in an attempt to find a solution to the malaria problem for it is known that people living in malaria endemic areas develop some limited natural immunity to malaria. This naturally acquired immunity appears to be very limited and may be very specific to a type of malaria. Research work indicates that this limited immunity quickly disappears when an individual moves away from the endemic area for some time.

This discovery that the body can develop some natural immunity to malaria is the basis for the current research to develop a vaccine against malaria. Several universities and research institutions are currently putting some efforts in this direction.

Based on the assumption that such efforts could be rewarded with success, the PATH Malaria Vaccine initiative (MVI) was set up in 1999 through a grant from the Bill and Melinda Gates Foundation. Its mission was to identify potentially promising vaccine candidates and systematically move them through the development stage and ensure that countries which need them most will be ready to use them as soon as they are available.

A major landmark of this effort is 2015 when a licensed, first generation malaria vaccine with at least 50% efficacy against severe disease for at least one year should be available.

Another public–private sector business entity that is working to develop and market malaria drugs is the Swiss based company called Medicines for Malaria Ventures (MMV). This company which also receives public and private sector grants does research with several universities in the Northern hemisphere. It is sad to note that none of these organizations have research collaboration with universities and scientific research centers in Africa.

The sterilization of male mosquitoes by ionizing radiation

The idea of sterilizing male mosquitoes has been around since the discovery and generalization of methods of irradiation in several areas of industry. Mosquito irradiation methods are based on the idea of breeding and then sterilizing large numbers of male mosquitoes with ionizing radiation and then releasing them into the wild with the hope that these sterile mosquitoes would mate with their female counterparts, resulting in the production of sterile eggs. Since these eggs would be incapable of hatching to produce viable mosquitoes, the mosquito populations would significantly diminish to levels that would wipe them out of any ecosystem. To date, very little information is available on the laboratory research and field work in this area.

CHEMICAL CONTROL METHODS

...the use of insecticides --generalized spraying

Many countries have a generalized national insecticide spray program. An insecticide called dichloro-diphenyl-trichloroethane (DDT) was synthesized by a German Chemistry student in 1874. However its effective use as a formidable insecticide was not known until in 1939 when the discovery was made by a Swiss scientist called Paul Muller. In the years that followed this discovery, especially from 1942 to 1945 and afterwards, DDT was used all over the world to kill mosquitoes. Due to its effectiveness, the World Health Organization in 1955, proposed a program to the World health Assembly to eradicate malaria from the world once and for all. To this effect, DDT was combined with new anti-malarials especially chloroquine in a 4 step program to achieve this goal. These steps were: preparation, attack, consolidation and maintenance. The development of chloroquine resistant malaria parasites and the discovery of toxic side effects of DDT in North America were a few of the reasons that led the failure of the program and its abandonment. Other reasons included the exclusion of sub-Saharan African countries from the program and the lack of community participation in many areas.

In spite of the failure of this global initiative however, many countries have a national insecticide spraying program which accompanies national malaria control programs. Depending on the type of chemical, most insecticides provide best results when they are applied in small droplets between 10 and 100 microns in size. This is most cost effective especially in enclosed areas and places with limited wind.

In places where there is wind, insecticides diffused in this size range end up being carried away to long distances, far away from where they are most needed. Therefore, in places where there is uncontrolled wind, insecticide spraying machines are made to deliver chemical products as droplets between 200 to 400 microns in size. Their heavier sizes make them less easily transportable by wind. In this way, the sprayed insecticide droplets tend to stay around the areas where they are needed.

Two methods of spraying are often used in mosquito control programs. These are –**Thermal fogging** spraying and –**Cold fogging [also called Ultra–low volume (ULV)]** spraying.

The **Thermal fogging method** employs devices that use heat to produce a fog without any degradation to the chemical insecticide. Thermal foggers produce droplets in many, widely varying sizes including several droplets with very small sizes. The varied sizes of the drops help create a fog where the insecticide has been sprayed. The thermal fogging method is the method of choice for areas of dense vegetation or areas with obstructions like city buildings. In addition, the visible nature of the fog produced helps the Spraying-Technician to monitor progress and to differentiate between treated and non-treated areas.

An **Ultra-low volume spray method** produces droplets of a more precise nature. It does this by employing high volume air at reduced pressure. However, the precise calibration of droplet size that the cold fog method allows enables these sprayers to dispense insecticides in more condensed formulations. Furthermore, they allow chemicals to be dispensed in the exact droplet size required to produce the most effective results.

Environmental Protection Agencies in several countries regulate the use of insecticides due to toxic effects on the environment. EPA recommended insecticides are therefore regarded as relatively safe and as environmentally friendly as possible. Current EPA allowed insecticides include resmethrin, permethrin and natural pyrethrin.

...the use of insecticide repellents: mosquito coils and sprays

Mosquito coils and aerosol sprays are by far the most widely used household mosquito insecticides in Asia and Africa. They are relatively inexpensive and easily available in local markets. An estimated seven billion coils are sold each year in Indonesia alone. In Africa and Asia, people burn mosquito coils in their sleeping rooms while sleeping at night to ward off attacks by mosquitoes. These people expose themselves to chemical and smoke inhalation from the coils during this time. However, these coils barely kill mosquitoes. At best, they render some mosquitoes temporarily inactive.

Mosquito coils are made from pyrethroids, which are common household insecticides. Pyrethroids are of two types:

Pyrethroid Type 1 also called **Allethrin** is the type used in mosquito coil manufacture. Allethrin has no cyano group and acts on sodium channels causing repetitive discharges in nerve fibers thus leading to hyper-excitation in humans.

Pyrethroid Type 2 (deltamethrin, fenvalerate) is more toxic and can cause nerve membrane depolarization as well as nerve membrane block leading to paralysis. It is generally not used in mosquito coil manufacture.

Pyrethroid Type 1 (Allethrin) poisoning can led to ataxia, loss of coordination, hyper-excitation and convulsions. However, the human system of metabolism rapidly converts allethrin by ester hydrolysis and hydroxylation to their inactive acids and alcohol components making them relatively safe products. The fatal dose for allethrin is not known. Deaths from allethrin have been reported in cases when convulsions increase in duration and do not stop within 2-3 weeks
No specific antidote is known for either Pyrethroid Type 1 or Type 2 poisoning.

However, pyrethroids may not be the only compounds found in mosquito coils. Mosquito coil manufacture practices vary in different countries and this may be cause for alarm.

Recently a study by Robert Krieger, Travis Dinoff and Xiaofei Zhang of the Department of Entomology, University of California, Riverside revealed that Indonesian mosquito coils and Chinese made ones imported into Southern California contained S-2 (octachlorodipropyl ether), a known lung carcinogen.

Due to the widely used nature of these coils, some researchers have called for studies to find an acceptable formulation for mosquito coils until safer controls in manufacturing practices are widely accepted. To buttress this call, the WHO organization, in 1998 called for research to determine safe levels of exposure to S-2 from mosquito coils. Up to now, no known research has been done to this effect.

..... the use of skin repellents eg. DEET

Skin repellents are chemical substances that humans smear on their bodies to discourage mosquitoes from feeding on their exposed skins. They are toxic to mosquitoes and repel them when they approach a human victim to feed. Skin repellents offer limited protection, usually varying from one to two hours. In order to prolong the effectiveness of skin repellents, some formulas provide sustained release or controlled release products. Such products provide longer lasting effects.

Skin repellents are commercially available as aerosols, creams or liquids. The following are some of the effective insect repellents.

DEET: The most widely used of these skin repellents is DEET (N, N-diethyl-3-methylbenzamide or N,N-diethyl-mtoluamide). It is best to avoid applying DEET concentrations of more than 30% to any human skin, particularly to those of children. Repellents should also not be applied to the eyes, noses, lips, irritated or broken skin. DEET is available commercially in 7% concentrations. Commercially available DEET containing insect repellents include *Off, Cutter, Ultrathon and Sawyer.*

Picaridin: Another known skin repellent is Picaridin whose chemical name is 2-(2-hydroxyethyl)-1-piperidinecarboxylic acid 1-methylpropyl ester. Picaridin is found in commercial products like *Cutter advanced, Skin-so-soft, Bug Guard Plus* and *Autan.* Picaridin is commercially available in 15% concentrations and may be applied directly to human skin to offer protection from mosquito bites.

PMD or Oil of Lemon Eucalyptus: PMD or oil of lemon eucalyptus is a synthetic version of lemon eucalyptus. Its chemical name is para-menthane-3-8-diol. It is commercially available as *Repel.*

Repellents which contain permethrin are useless when applied to human skin. Permethrin containing products are very useful insecticides when applied to clothing, shoes, bed nets and window curtains. Permethrin treated clothes retain their effectiveness even after the clothes or curtains have been washed many times.

Chapter 8:	ERADICATION OF MALARIA

Malaria control versus malaria eradication

There is no doubt that the scourge of malaria must be eradicated. To do this effectively, the parasite responsible for the disease must be eliminated and mosquito carriers of the disease must be destroyed. Research data suggest that the major question is not whether humanity has the human and technical resources to accomplish this, but whether there is the social and political will to do it. Available data point to the fact that countries with the correct social and political will have eradicated malaria.

.....have some countries have succeeded in eradicating malaria? YES!!!!

Countries which have succeeded in eradicating malaria include Italy, Portugal, Spain, the Netherlands and the USA. Others include Yugoslavia, Romania, Bulgaria, Hungary and Czechoslovakia. Even the North African countries of Algeria, Morocco, Tunisia and Libya are reported to be free of malaria though the risk of the disease is not completely absent because the possibility of imported malaria still exist.

Malaria control is not malaria eradication. Malaria control aims at reducing the incidence of malaria, bringing down the horrible statistics of death and disease on an annual basis. It aims at pest source reduction including some very limited control over the number of infections and human deaths. Malaria control does not aim at eliminating malaria completely.

On the other hand, malaria eradication means the complete elimination of the malaria disease from a particular environment. It aims at the total destruction and eradication of the various parasites that are responsible for the disease. If in doing so, the mosquito pest is eliminated, that would also be a very welcome addition. This is because even in the absence of the parasite, the mosquito continuously harasses people in warm climates all the year round and those in temperate climates during the warm seasons of the year. For example, in North America, where malaria has been eradicated, those who attempt to stay outdoors at dawn or at dusk are pestered unceasingly by painful mosquito bites, especially during the warm months of the year.

How will eradication be successfully accomplished?
Numerous approaches to reducing mosquito populations through pest source reduction exist. These have been described in an earlier chapter and include:
  -physical control methods
  -biological control methods
  -chemical control methods
Some approaches to eliminating the *Plasmodium* parasites responsible for malaria from its human host also exist. These include:
  -use of medication to destroy the parasite in patients (treatment of infected patients)
  -use of medication to prevent the parasite from developing in patients (prophylaxis)

-the search for vaccines against the parasite

Current research results for a vaccine against malaria is showing some promise but there is not any adequate vaccine yet. The year 2015 has been projected as the time when a vaccine should be ready for trials. In the meantime therefore, for malaria eradication to be successful, vector control methods and infected human treatment methods must be employed on a simultaneous basis. These two approaches, working together, must constitute an important step in an effective comprehensive program targeted to an individual community. At the same time, structures must be put into place to enable the mobilization of political, social and economic structures towards meeting eradication goals within specific geographic areas. For any program to be successful, each of these two steps should be considered as important as the other and be mutually dependent. How would these two entities be interwoven to meet goals for successful eradication in developing countries, especially those in sub-Saharan Africa? Before we answer that question, let us look at lessons learned from the failed malaria eradication program in the later part of the 1950s.

...lessons from the failed malaria eradication project in the 1950's

In the period following the Second World War, DDT was discovered to be a very effective insecticide. Coupled with the discovery of new anti-malarial drugs like chloroquine, the World Health Organization proposed a four stage program to the World Health Assembly to rid the world of the scourge of malaria. The project included insecticide spraying of dwelling places, the distribution of anti-malarial drugs for malaria treatment purposes and surveillance. The program achieved some success. Malaria was eradicated in several countries that had temperate climates and also in places where malaria was seasonal. In other countries like India and Sri Lanka, there were very significant reductions in malaria infections. However, in the early 1960's, environmentalists started drawing attention to the toxic effects of DDT in North America. In addition, chloroquine resistant parasites were discovered in some countries. Environmental groups brought pressure to bear on the malaria eradication program and it was abandoned.

The abandonment of the project and its consequent failure led to the re-emergence of malaria in India and Sri Lanka. It should be pointed out that the program achieved negligible results in places like Haiti, Afghanistan, Indonesia and Nicaragua. Some researchers say that the lack of community involvement in many places contributed to its failure. Other major factors often cited for the failure of the project include large population migrations, wars, political and social factors as well as difficulties in obtaining funding for its long term goals. Worst of all, the most malaria endemic countries in the world like sub-Saharan Africa were left out of the project.

Incorporating vector control

The numerous physical, biological and chemical control methods used in controlling the mosquito pest are outlined in an earlier chapter and are as follows:

Physical control methods

- environmental destruction and elimination of breeding sites
- the use of bed-nets at night to prevent mosquito feeding on humans
- the use of mosquito screens to protect all house entrances
- the use of catch-and-destroy traps

Biological control methods

- the use of natural predators to control adult mosquitoes and larvae
- the use of artificially introduced bacteria to kill mosquito larvae
- the use of sound energy to destroy larvae
- the development of an effective vaccine
- sterilization of male mosquitoes by ionizing irradiation

Chemical control methods

- the use of insecticides
- the use of larvicides
- the use of skin products that discourage mosquito feeding on humans eg DEET
- the use of non-skin contact repellents like mosquito coils, pyrethroids,

Vector Control: Incorporating physical control methods

With determination, it is possible to destroy and eliminate all mosquito breeding sites in any developing country. Even without the use of insecticides, mosquito breeding sites and mosquitoes were eliminated in Cuba during the early part of the 19th century by US forces which were stationed there. A combined effort of water drainage and oil treatment of remaining pools and puddles on a consistent basis achieved these enviable results. The same can be done anywhere. Many developing countries use an open drain system which is made up of open gutters that are often full of weeds and stagnant water. This system must be changed in favor of closed drains. A system of closed drains will not allow growing weeds or stagnant water that will favor mosquito breeding. Remaining large open bodies of stagnant water can be dealt with using the new arsenal of larvicides.

Empowered by US President George Bush's Presidential Malaria Initiative (PMI), insecticide-treated bed-nets started to be distributed in 15 African countries to help reduce the transmission of malaria by preventing mosquito bites. These efforts will need to be sustained. The production of new insecticide treated bed nets with long lasting effects against mosquitoes (some Manufacturers say they can last 8 years of washing and use) is a welcome addition to the continuously growing arsenal against malaria.

It is difficult to evaluate how many people in developing countries can afford to screen their dwelling places against mosquitoes, but a large number of city dwellers in many African countries have mosquito screened porches and rooms. As the economies of these countries continue to improve, and technology lowers the cost of plastics, it is possible that this trend will continue. On the other hand, with the low price of cotton, many developing countries can use locally produced cotton to manufacture bed-nets that can be insecticide-treated and then used by the local population.

By far, the use of catch and destroy traps may play a substantial role in mosquito eradication. Today, a large number of catch and destroy traps are available. These vary from some very simple ones to very elaborate ones that employ modern, sophisticated technology. Indications are high that these catch-and-destroy traps equally vary in the numbers and types of mosquitoes they can catch and destroy. If catch-and-destroy traps must be used in an effective malaria eradication program in developing countries, then it must be possible for local artisans to manufacture them from locally available materials at a very low and affordable cost to the local population. Local research to adapt existing trap manufacture to local conditions of production and use must be vigorously pursued and the results implemented without delay.

When these traps are produced by local artisans and used at the village level, it should be possible to mobilize school children to take an active interest in them and supervise their performance on a weekly basis. Local competitions to evaluate performance of improved traps and mosquito catch numbers should stimulate interest in these traps and facilitate their continuous use.

Available research shows that the more sophisticated traps catch more mosquitoes. It stands to reason that the more attractants employed, the stronger will be the lure of mosquitoes and probably the higher the catch. Many developing nations have local electric and electronic technicians who can be taught to manufacture these modern, sophisticated catch-and-destroy traps. And there are many households in developing nations with the financial ability to purchase these traps. Again, methods of production of these traps must be adequately researched and adapted to local needs. It must be emphasized that these traps must be produced by local entrepreneurs so that problems of after sales maintenance can be resolved adequately and rapidly within the local environment.

It will be very important for local governments to create the necessary financial and commercial national support for those private companies that will like to venture into this domain. The market is there and should be explored. Even, should government subsidies be necessary, such subsidies should be promptly allocated and disbursed, in view of the tremendous amount of benefits and savings that governments will make from a population living in a malaria free society.

Vector Control: Incorporating biological control methods

We should remember from an earlier chapter that biological control methods include the following:

- the use of natural predators to control adult mosquitoes and larvae
- the use of larvicides (bacteria spores to kill mosquito larvae)
- the use of sound energy to destroy larvae
- the development of an effective vaccine
- sterilization of male mosquitoes by ionizing irradiation

Biological control methods have made gigantic strides in recent years. The use of fish eating mosquitoes and frogs may be limited but it can be encouraged. Mosquito-eating fish could provide much needed protein in many malnourished areas. However, two recently discovered methods stand out and hold a lot of promise. The first is the discovery and use of *Bacillus thuringensis israelensis* (bti) and *Bacillus sphaericus* spores to destroy larvae in stagnant water. With these larvicides, mosquito larvae could be easily eliminated from large bodies of water in very short periods of time and such bodies of water maintained mosquito free for several years with the continuous sprinkling of bacteria spores on the water surface. Limited application of this method in Ghana quite recently resulted in massive drops of mosquito numbers and infections (up to 68%) in a 6 month period. Efforts should be made to produce these bacteria in developing countries. Again the technology for the industrial production of these bacteria spores is within the grasp of many developing African countries. For instance, there is hardly any African country that does not produce drinking beer. And anybody in fermentation technology would know that the production of these bacteria closely resembles the modern-day industrial production of drinking beer. Wherever possible, Bacillus spore production under license with partners in industrialized countries should ensure mutual benefits to patent-holders and industrial producers in developing countries.

The second most important development in biological vector control is the discovery that sound waves can destroy mosquito larvae. This technology also holds great promise. Again, local research of this technology should be adequately pursued to find how best to adapt it to local needs.

Efforts to develop an effective vaccine against malaria infections are under way. The sad thing is that none of this research is taking place in developing African countries. This anomaly should be rectified. Scientific and research institutions should be mandated and funded to join in the search for a malaria vaccine. It is good to know that philanthropic donors like the Bill and Melinda Gates Foundation are providing substantial, unrestricted grants to many research centers doing malaria research. Developing countries should mobilize graduate universities and research centers to pursue some of these grants aggressively in order to undertake serious fundamental and applied research in malaria.

There is not much published practical application data on the irradiation of mosquitoes and their use in malaria eradication. This method of malaria vector control has therefore not been tried and tested on a large scale. However, this area holds promise for those countries with a nuclear agenda. Developing countries with rudimentary nuclear medicine facilities like Ghana could probably take a lead in this direction.

Vector Control: Incorporating chemical control methods

We have discussed chemical control methods in an earlier chapter. These include:
- the use of insecticides
- the use of larvicides
- the use of skin products that discourage mosquito feeding on humans eg DEET
- the use of non-skin contact repellents like mosquito coils, pyrethroids

Chemical control methods have always formed the backbone of any program geared towards malaria eradication. This is because industrialized countries have adequate control over the production, sales and distribution over chemical substances. This method is therefore often sold to developing countries as an affordable and reliable method of pest eradication. Although mass spraying can, and has been used to achieve low pest populations in many developing countries, they hardly constitute a panacea to the problem of pest eradication in developing countries. For one, developing countries hardly produce any chemical insecticides and therefore need to import these chemicals in large quantities. This often strains national budgets. Secondly, many insects develop resistance to insecticides pretty quickly, especially when used inappropriately and in environments and cultures which have hardly been the subjects of thorough scientific enquiry. Thirdly, many chemicals have toxic effects on non target flora and fauna including humans.

In spite of these objections, when insecticides are appropriately combined with other methods or pest eradication, they could provide immediate substantial reduction in mosquito numbers. An initial heavy dose of a long lasting insecticide application combined with several vector reduction methods could provide a 'blitzkrieg' approach that would instantly reduce mosquito numbers substantially. This could then open the way for a sustained elimination program to keep mosquito numbers below its population survival levels and gradually lead to malaria disease eradication.

.........Incorporating political, social and economic factors

Political, social and economic factors are by far the most formidable obstacles to the eradication of malaria in developing countries. Many politicians in developing countries can hardly boast of any meaningful short, medium or long term plans for national development. If they did, malaria eradication would be the first on the agenda, for an unhealthy population can hardly help local governments to attain economic and political independence goals. It is a truism that in many developing countries, political leaders, structures and parties determine almost everything, from life to death. It can therefore be said that, it is these political leaders who make a program succeed or who spell its doom. If there is political will, social conditions and structures can be easily mobilized towards a defined goal and make it succeed. It therefore stands to reason, that malaria eradication in any developing country should start with the blatant seduction of the country's political machinery for its total cooperation. The resources of the Ministry of Health should be borrowed, acquired and transformed to help play a major role in the malaria eradication program. Major establishments like the military, para-military forces, political parties, college students and the unemployed should be mobilized in this direction. International political pressure should be brought to bear on insensitive political leaders. In a loud and clear manner, all the financial and health benefits that can accrue to the nation should be spelt out to both politicians and the local population on a continuous and regular basis.

In addition to political institutions, two main social structures may be called upon to play a meaningful role in malaria eradication programs. These are:

-Traditional institutions

-Faith-based institutions

Many countries in Sub-Saharan Africa still have traditional institutions that play well defined roles in the lives of the local population. For instance, in many parts of Africa, it is the traditional social and political institutions that determine when annual festivals must be held. The traditional institutions are also responsible for enforcing traditional and customary rules and regulations within the ethnic boundaries. The Chiefs and Elders of these traditional institutions also serve as spiritual and religious leaders and links between the ancestors and the living. In spite of modern day political institutions and political parties, these traditional leaders are of significant importance to the members of the different ethnic groups they are supposed to serve. It is therefore important that these traditional leaders be informed and their cooperation sought in any malaria eradication project. Such traditional political structures, however rudimentary, could then be mobilized with the help of the traditional institutions to help in the malaria eradication program.

Traditional religions, Christianity and Islam are the three main religious practices in Africa. The roles that traditional political and religious institutions should play have been discussed. Africans who shy away from traditional political and religious practices in daylight are often found in churches and mosques. Church pastors and Muslim leaders should therefore be adequately informed about malaria eradication programs and their full blessings and cooperation obtained. Christian pastors and ministers can mobilize their members during church services and inform them of the project. They can also organize seminars and education programs to dispense information about the project, seek input, monitor effectiveness and ensure success. Islamic leaders can do likewise in mosques on Fridays and dispense vital information and ask for cooperation from worshippers.

It is very important to stress that political and social leaders must be approached in a respectful way. The ideals and the goals of the malaria eradication program should be carefully explained to them and their full blessings obtained. An attitude of superciliousness and arrogance towards these institutions should be avoided at all costs. The project should be seen as a collaborative effort geared towards the benefit of all. Success stories should be shared and failures analyzed properly with the view to finding ways to ensure success. However, the financial and economic resources for the malaria eradication program should never be put under the management of any of these institutions.

Management of Malaria Eradication Agencies

In view of the importance that should be attached to this project, it is imperative that malaria management agencies be removed from the umbrella of government bureaucracy. Malaria eradication programs should have a supra-national authority and have both independent national and international supervision. Such organizations should be mandated to have as their priority the total eradication of malaria within the shortest possible time. The following are a few of the goals that should be set for any malaria eradication agency that hopes to achieve its goal.

Such organizations should be able:
-to discover the most appropriate methods of achieving malaria eradication goals

-to mobilize local populations on the need to achieve the goals of malaria eradication

-to explain distinctly to the local population the difference between malaria control and   malaria eradication

-to define the most appropriate vector control methods and provide the required tools for   their application

-to help train local health authorities on all aspects of the project

-to help in the insecticide diffusion program

-to train local artisans on the manufacture, sale and after sale servicing of mosquito traps

-to help in the distribution and acquisition of such traps by individuals

-to monitor the spread of larvicides or other agents on water bodies

-to monitor any such vector control methods and provide quantifiable results

-to work closely with national and international agencies with similar goals

-to present to national and international agencies the obstacles likely to lead to failure and   provide advice on how to remove any such obstacles

-to work assiduously towards achieving the goals of malaria eradication within the   shortest possible time.

And when all the initials goals have been attained, the agencies should be transformed into watchdogs of malaria surveillance, control and eradication.

Chapter 9 : Social and Economic importance of malaria eradication

Statistics compiled by the World Health Organization indicate that about 350 – 500 million cases of malaria infections are reported in the world each year. Of these reported infectious episodes, between 0.7 – 2.7 million patients die every year. Some 3.2 billion people living in 107 countries are at risk because they live in malaria transmission areas. Even in countries where malaria has been eradicated, public health officials are forced to maintain constant surveillance by spending considerable human, technical and financial resources to keep mosquito populations down and guard against the re-introduction of malaria. In many developing countries, malaria continuously saps the health of individuals, rendering them weak and sick on a perpetual basis. Living with this scourge robs millions of people and several nations of valuable financial resources necessary for personal and national development, maintaining many of them in a vicious cycle of poverty and deprivation. The situation is particularly acute in developing countries especially sub-Saharan Africa where malaria is the leading cause of death and disease due to warmer temperatures and a particularly virulent malaria parasite.

This is unacceptable.

In spite of this, current thinking on malaria as exemplified by the **World's Roll Back Malaria Program** aims at malaria control. However, malaria control is not malaria eradication. The objective of malaria control is to reduce the levels of malaria infection to "previously decided acceptable levels" and not to eradicate the disease. Seen in this context therefore, the objective of the World's Roll Back Program malaria control program is to reduce by half the burden of malaria infections and death by the year 2010. Even with conservative estimates, this would still mean the world living with and accepting malaria deaths ranging from 0.4 – 1.4 million annually with 175-250 million infectious cases and deaths of about 0.4–1.4 million each year. Without substantial efforts at national and international levels, it is doubtful that even these mediocre goals of malaria control will be met in several developing countries. It is possible to do better. It is possible to aim higher. Humanity can and should strive to eradicate malaria. Malaria must be eradicated in order to bring hope and the promise of a better life to billions of poor people living with this scourge in over 100 countries of the world.

........has malaria been eradicated in some countries? YES!!!

Several countries have been able to eradicate malaria. Notable among these are the United States, Portugal, France, Italy, Holland, Hungary, Poland, Canada and Scandinavian countries.

...is malaria eradication possible in developing nations? Yes!!!

As has already been noted in an earlier chapter, many industrialized countries have been able to eradicate malaria. But is malaria eradication also possible in developing countries? The North African countries of Algeria, Tunisia and Libya are developing countries. These countries may be favored by cold winter temperatures that help reduce mosquito populations, but it is a fact that when temperatures soar during the spring, summer and autumn months, there are hardly any reported cases of malaria outbreaks. Even, the island of Seychelles which is found off the coast of Tropical Africa, hardly reports any cases of malaria outbreaks. So, without a doubt, malaria can be eradicated in developing countries.

.....malaria eradication will bring riches to developing countries..

In 2007, the Ghanaian Minister for Health, Courage Quashigah announced that his country recorded 30 million cases of malaria that year and that the country spent 777 million dollars on malaria treatment. It should be pointed out that in such a developing country where a large number of people do not have access to hospital facilities, this figure does not include individual spending on self-diagnosis and self-treatment. It equally does not take into account losses in national revenue due to absenteeism and substantially decreased productivity by suffering sick and feeble workers. The actual total financial burden of malaria on the Ghanaian economy is far more than that reported by the Minister of Health and may never be known. This would make the UNICEF estimate of over 2 billion dollars being the financial costs of malaria to Sub-Saharan African countries largely under-estimated. With over 43 independent African countries, the total financial losses may well be in the region of over 30 – 40 billion dollars.

An attempt to analyze this important loss of revenue would divide financial losses from malaria infections into 2 main categories:

-costs to individuals

-costs to government

...costs to individuals

In many developing countries, malaria patients may go to nearby hospitals for treatment. Whereas most malaria patients are seen as out-patients, and sent home after receiving the necessary prescription, some patients with serious cases of malaria infection end up being admitted in the hospitals for observation and treatment. Surveys undertaken in several parts of Ghana show that in a typical hospital, 3 out of 10 beds may be occupied at any time by malaria patients.

In cases where hospitals are far away, patients often indulge in self-diagnosis and self-treatment. Treatment methods vary considerably and vary from the use of local herbs to chloroquine based pharmaceuticals and other concoctions sold in local drug stores.

The costs to an individual infected patient may therefore include the following:

-Cost of travel to the health center or doctor's office or to purchase drugs

-costs from consultation with a health provider or doctor

-costs due to drug purchases

-costs from lost days of work and revenue

–costs to protect oneself from mosquitoes and malaria infection, for example, mosquito coils, bed nets, window screens, insecticides sprays (aerosols) and

–in the case of death, funeral expenses and responsibility of orphans

These costs are hardly quantified and reported in national statistical surveys.

–

...costs to governments

In 2006, the Ministry of Health in Ghana reported that malaria represented 88.9% of the total annual medical consultations of diseases that cannot be prevented by vaccination. Like in many developing countries, most responsibility for health care rests with the government and traditional doctors. However, it is the Ministry and health care departments who build clinics and health care centers, employ and pay the salaries of doctors, nurses and staff.

It is also the Ministry that imports or purchases drugs for the treatment of diseases like malaria. Governments in developing countries are also often the major employer of the country's citizens. Absenteeism due to illnesses and low productivity due to sick and feeble working adults also affect government business adversely. Therefore, governments bear a large brunt of the responsibility that goes with a sick and weak population living in a malaria endemic area. A list of costs of malaria to governments will include:

The costs of malaria infections to governments include
–costs of building health care centers

-costs of payment of salaries for doctors, nurses and other health workers

-costs of drug imports

-costs of drugs purchased from local manufacturers

-costs of health education

-costs of imports of insecticides and /or physical agents against mosquito bites, mosquito coils, bed-nets, mosquito screens

-costs of purchase and spraying of insecticides

-costs due to loss in revenue from worker absenteeism and low productivity from a feeble and /or sick working population

-costs due to loss of potential international joint business ventures

-costs from loss in tourism due to potential tourists' fear of contracting malaria.

It is evident that a sick and unhealthy population will have little to contribute in way of innovation and planning for a better future for the individuals and the nation. It is therefore not surprising to learn that it is estimated that there is loss of growth on 1.3% in the economies off malaria endemic countries as compared to those without malaria.

...tolerating malaria, a question of misplaced priorities...

It seems obvious that the inability of governments on developing countries to provide adequate malaria control and/or its complete eradication is one of misplaced priorities and lack of political will at the governmental level. To explain this in more detail, let us look at a simple statistical analysis of the situation in one developing country, Ghana.

Former US President George Bush's initiative to provide treated mosquito nets to developing countries was able to provide treated bed-nets at US5.00 a piece through a public-private initiative called *Malaria-No-More* (MNM) organization. If the Ghanaian government had provided these bed-nets to its 22 million people, it would have spent 110 million to provide a net for every single Ghanaian. Better still, using locally produced cotton wool from local farms to provide bed-nets and subsequently treating them with imported (or locally produced pyrethroids) would have resulted in many employment opportunities for Ghanaians and substantial savings to the country.

Such a project would have eliminated more than half of the cases of malaria in the country resulting in at least 50% savings for its Ministry of Health. Rather, in the same year 2007, the Ghanaian government chose to embark on the building of a palace for its President at a cost of 138 million dollars. The following year, 2008, it again spent 760 million dollars on malaria treatment.

Year	Expenditure on Malaria treatment	Estimated Bed-Net cost for whole population	Estimated Govt. savings
2007	777 million	5 x 22 m = 110 m	777-110 = 667 m
2008	760 million	5x 22m = 110m	760-110 = 650 m

Table 9-1: Simple analysis of estimated savings in US dollars from the supply of bed-nets to every Ghanaian in 2007 and 2008 (estimated Ghanaian population 22 million).

This analysis may be simplistic, but even if the expenditure on malaria treatment was cut in half, this would amount to a savings of well over 300 million dollars to the Ghanaian government for that year alone. And that does not include the increase in national productivity that would have resulted from a healthy, malaria-free population.

Conclusion

Malaria brings untold hardship and suffering to millions of people. Mosquitoes collect blood from human beings to feed their eggs and bring to life a healthy offspring to the detriment of human children. By so doing, mosquito offspring live, while we and our children die. This is unacceptable. Malaria can and must be eradicated from the developing countries. This will bring prosperity, good health and happiness to millions of people and needy governments. The time for action is now.

Remember, that it is the life of a human baby and yours, or that of the mosquito.

Enough is enough. The time for action is NOW. Please, help eradicate malaria now.

Remember:
NO MOSQUITO   NO MALARIA.
KNOW THE MOSQUITO. KNOW MALARIA.
FEED THE MOSQUITO. FEED MALARIA.
FEED THE MOSQUITO. KILL THE CHILD
FEED THE MOSQUITO. KILL YOURSELF!

REFERENCES and READINGS OF INTEREST

1. Africa Fighting Malaria AFM document 2008

2. Centers for Disease Control report. The Impact of Malaria– A leading cause of Death Worldwide. See also Control and Prevention, Diagnosis and Treatment, Disease, Epidemiology, Geographic Distribution, History. CDC Atlanta. GA USA   in

3. DDT: wikipedia The free encyclopedia. http://en.wikipedia.org/wiki/ddt

4. Global Defence against the Infectious Disease Threat. WHO Report 2003

5. Krieger R., Travis Duff Zhang Xiaofei report on Mosquito Coils by Brandon Adams. Environmental Health Sciences www.ehponline.org

6. Malaria, Anopheles mosquitoes CDC report Division of Parasitic Diseases (last   modified Sept 7 2004)

7. Malaria: ECOWAS to adopt Ghana Measures Ghana News Agency Report March 29   2009.

8. Malaria NO MORE Report, 2008

9. Malaria: What is malaria. Medicine for Malaria Ventures (MMV) Annual Report 2007. Geneva, Switzerland.

10. Nelson R, Jackson R. *Evarcha culicivora* University of Canterbury, Christchurch, New Zealand. Report by Charles Q. Choi, Live Science, January 14, 2007

11. Plasmodium falciparum biology in Plasmodium falciparum biology. Modified 20th July 2008 http://en.wikipedia.org/Plasmodium

12. US President's Malaria Initiative report 2008

13. Prinalgin: Yellow Fever: Its five phases and its History in America. Jan 10 2007

14. Tom Floore, Public Health Entomology Research and Education center, Florida, USA

15. UNICEF: United Nations Children' Fund. Report on malaria 2005

16. WHO World Malaria Report 2005

17. World Health Organization www.who.int/topics/malaria

18. Yellow Fever: Chemical and Biological Warfare Information. In Chemical and Biological Weapons for Emergency Safety and Security Personnel. 1999

See also the following internet sites:

www.stopmalarianow.net site for Stop Malaria Now Foundation, Morrow, United States and Accra, Ghana.

www.stopmalariaAfrica.org site for Stop Malaria Now Foundation, Morrow, United States and Accra, Ghana.

www.malarianomore.org site for Malaria No More Organization

www.MMV.com site for Medicine for Malaria Ventures, Switzerland.

www.Africafightingmalaria.com site for Africa Fighting Malaria Organization.

www.fightingmalaria.gov site for President Bush's Malaria Initiative Organization

www.CDC.gov/malaria site for the United States Centers for Disease Control (CDC), Atlanta.

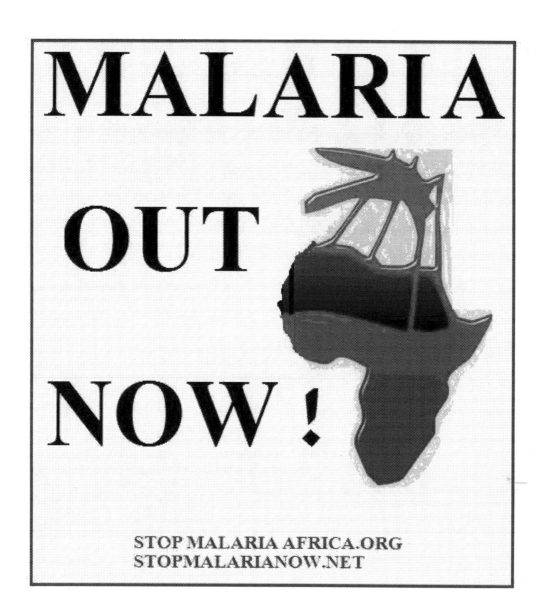

STOP MALARIA AFRICA.ORG
STOPMALARIANOW.NET